Fibroids and Reproduction

Fibroids and Reproduction

Edited by

Botros R.M.B. Rizk, MD, MA, FRCOG, FRCS, HCLD, FACOG, FACS

Medical Director, Elite IVF, Houston, Texas
Medical Director, Advanced Fertility Centers
Odessa Fertility Lab Director
Odessa, Texas
President, Middle East Fertility Society
Adjunct Professor of Obstetrics and Gynecology
Cairo University Medical School
and Department of Obstetrics and Gynecology
Kasr El Eini Hospital
Cairo, Egypt
Formerly Professor and Head, Reproductive Endocrinology and Infertility
University of South Alabama, Mobile, Alabama

Yakoub Khalaf, MBBCh, MSc, MD, FRCOG, MFFP

Professor of Reproductive Medicine and Surgery
Guy's and St Thomas' Hospital and King's College London
Head of Fertility Services and Director of the Assisted Conception Unit
and Centre for Pre-Implantation Genetic Diagnosis
Guy's and St Thomas' Hospital
London, United Kingdom

Mostafa A. Borahay, MD, PhD

Associate Professor of Gynecology and Obstetrics
Director of Minimally Invasive Gynecologic Surgery
Johns Hopkins Bayview Medical Center
Johns Hopkins University
Baltimore, Maryland

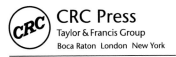

CRC Press
Taylor & Francis Group
Boca Raton London New York

CRC Press is an imprint of the
Taylor & Francis Group, an **informa** business

First edition published 2021
by CRC Press
6000 Broken Sound Parkway NW, Suite 300, Boca Raton, FL 33487-2742

and by CRC Press
2 Park Square, Milton Park, Abingdon, Oxon, OX14 4RN

© 2021 Taylor & Francis Group, LLC

CRC Press is an imprint of Taylor & Francis Group, LLC

ISBN: 978-0-367-55067-7 (pbk)
ISBN: 978-1-138-30542-7 (hbk)
ISBN: 978-0-203-72898-7 (ebk)

Typeset in Times LT Std
by Nova Techset Private Limited, Bengaluru & Chennai, India

Visit the Taylor & Francis Web site at
http://www.taylorandfrancis.com

and the CRC Press Web site at
http://www.crcpress.com

Contents

Preface

Dear Reader,

We put in your hands a book that covers all aspects of clinical evaluation and management of uterine fibroids. We put in a lot of effort to get it in the best possible form to help you help your patients. We hope you enjoy it, as we enjoyed putting it together.

Our deepest appreciation to our families. Without their support and dedication, we could not have completed it.

We would also like to acknowledge our dearest friends and colleagues who shared the journey with us and thank Drs. Mohamed Aboulghar, Gamal Serour, Hossam Abdalla, Shawky Badawy, and Fouad Sattar for decades of friendship and cooperation. We would also like to thank Robert Peden and the staff who worked on this book.

Botros R.M.B. Rizk
Yakoub Khalaf
Mostafa A. Borahay

Contributors

Shima Albasha
Reproductive Endocrinology and Infertility
Department of Obstetrics and Gynecology
Hamad Medical Corporation
Doha, Qatar

Mona Al Helou
Makassed General Hospital
American University of Beirut University Hospital
Beirut, Lebanon

Ayman Al-Hendy
Department of Surgery
University of Illinois at Chicago
Chicago, Illinois

Maria Facadio Antero
Division of Reproductive Endocrinology and
    Infertility
Department of Gynecology and Obstetrics
Johns Hopkins University
Baltimore, Maryland

Mohamed A. Bedaiwy
Division of Reproductive Endocrinology
    and Infertility
Department of Obstetrics and Gynecology
University of British Columbia
Vancouver, British Columbia, Canada

Mostafa A. Borahay
Department of Gynecology and Obstetrics
Johns Hopkins Bayview Medical Center
Johns Hopkins University
Baltimore, Maryland

Linda C. Chu
Russell H. Morgan Department of Radiology and
    Radiological Science
Johns Hopkins University
Baltimore, Maryland

Chantel I. Cross
Division of Reproductive Endocrinology
    and Infertility
Department of Gynecology and Obstetrics
Johns Hopkins University
Baltimore, Maryland

Eman A. Elgindy
Department of Obstetrics and Gynecology
University of Zagazig
Zagazig, Egypt

Hoda Elkafas
Department of Pharmacology
    and Toxicology
National Organization for Drug Control
    and Research (NODCAR)
Cairo, Egypt

and

Department of Surgery
University of Illinois at Chicago
Chicago, Illinois

Anja Frost
Department of Gynecology and Obstetrics
Johns Hopkins University
Baltimore, Maryland

Mounes Aliyari Ghasabeh
Russell H. Morgan Department
    of Radiology and Radiological Science
Johns Hopkins University
Baltimore, Maryland

Magdi Hanafi
Gynecology Department
Emory Saint Joseph's Hospital
Atlanta, Georgia

Candice P. Holliday
Division of Reproductive Endocrinology and
    Infertility
Department of Obstetrics and Gynecology
University of South Alabama
Mobile, Alabama

Ihab R. Kamel
Russell H. Morgan Department of Radiology and
    Radiological Science
Johns Hopkins University
Baltimore, Maryland

Yakoub Khalaf
Reproductive Medicine and Surgery
Guy's and St Thomas' Hospital and King's
    College London
and
Centre for Pre-Implantation Genetic Diagnosis
Guy's and St Thomas' Hospital
London, United Kingdom

Jacqueline Y. Maher
Division of Reproductive Endocrinology
    and Infertility
Department of Gynecology and Obstetrics
Johns Hopkins University
Baltimore, Maryland

Nicole Catherine Michel
Alabama College of Osteopathic Medicine
Dothan, Alabama

Kristin Patzkowsky
Department of Gynecology and Obstetrics
Johns Hopkins University
Baltimore, Maryland

Botros R.M.B. Rizk
Elite IVF
Houston, Texas

and

Advanced Fertility Centers
Odessa, Texas

Natasha K. Simula
Department of Obstetrics and Gynecology
University of British Columbia
Vancouver, British Columbia, Canada

Kamaria C. Cayton Vaught
Division of Reproductive Endocrinology
    and Infertility
Department of Gynecology and Obstetrics
Johns Hopkins University
Baltimore, Maryland

Harold Wu
Division of Minimally Invasive Gynecologic
    Surgery
Department of Gynecology and Obstetrics
Johns Hopkins University School of Medicine
Baltimore, Maryland

Qiwei Yang
Department of Surgery
University of Illinois at Chicago
Chicago, Illinois

1

Fibroids and Reproduction: A Bird's-Eye View

Botros R.M.B. Rizk, Candice P. Holliday, and Yakoub Khalaf

CONTENTS

Introduction

A fibroid (or leiomyoma) is a benign, monoclonal, smooth muscle tumor of the uterus, which usually presents as multiple lesions (Figure 1.1) but can occur as a single lesion (Figure 1.2). Fibroids are diagnosed in 20%–40% of women, generally after age 30 years, with a stable increase in incidence with increasing age [1]. This age-related increase in incidence of fibroids should be considered when looking into the relationship between fibroids and reproductive dysfunction (subfertility or miscarriage), as both are intimately age related.

Although it is biologically plausible and clinically evident that fibroids are associated with reproductive dysfunction (see Chapter 2), a cause-effect relationship has not been established.

Most symptomatic fibroids can be diagnosed clinically, but crucial clinical information can be obtained by one imaging modality or another.

Ultrasound is a noninvasive imaging modality that is well tolerated by patients, and it is a rather inexpensive way to obtain a relatively accurate assessment of fibroids within the pelvis (see Chapter 8). Assessing fibroid size and location can be beneficial for planning surgery or for monitoring changes in fibroids over time (Figures 1.3–1.5).

In some complex cases (multiple fibroids, previous surgery, and associated morbidities), magnetic resonance imaging (MRI) can provide additional valuable information that could help in planning surgery or guide the choice of alternative therapeutic approaches, such as the use of uterine artery embolization (UAE) or MRI-guided focused ultrasound (see Chapter 7).

Classification

When fibroids develop from the uterine wall but distort the uterine cavity, it is helpful to detail the degree of uterine cavity impingement (see Chapter 7) with the Wamsteker and de Blok classification [2]. Following are the types of fibroids:

- 0: 100% of the fibroid is pedunculated into the uterine cavity
- I: Greater than 50% of the fibroid is within the uterine cavity
- II: Less than 50% of the fibroid is within the uterine cavity (i.e., greater than 50% of the fibroid is within the myometrium)

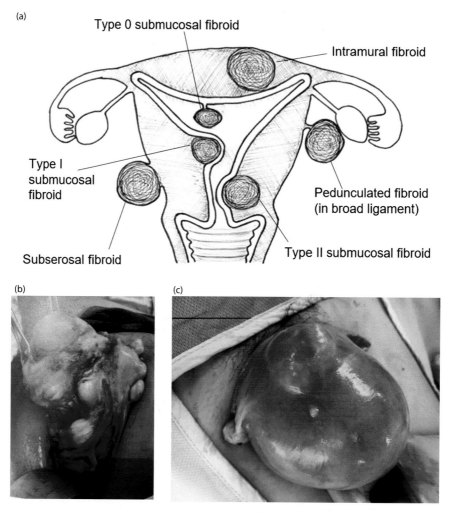

FIGURE 1.1   (a) Varying fibroid locations within the uterus; (b) multiple fibroids—intramural, subserosal, and submucosal; (c) uterus enlarged with intramural fibroids.

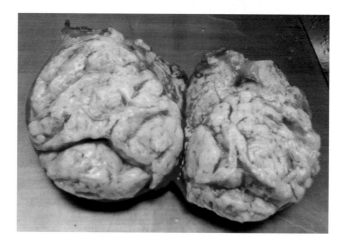

FIGURE 1.2   Solitary large fibroid.

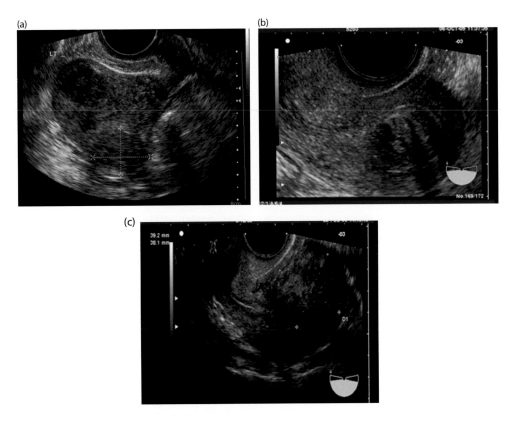

FIGURE 1.3 (a–c) Intramural fibroids.

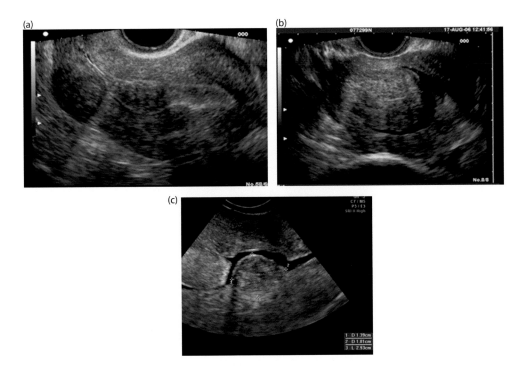

FIGURE 1.4 (a–c) Submucosal fibroids.

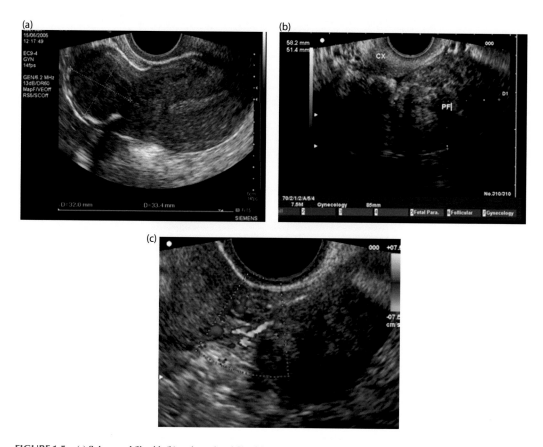

FIGURE 1.5   (a) Subserosal fibroid; (b) pedunculated fibroid; (c) Doppler scan showing feeder vessels of pedunculated fibroid.

It can be difficult to assess on two-dimensional (2D) ultrasound scan what type of fibroid a patient has. Three-dimensional (3D) ultrasound and saline infusion sonohysterography are often used to obtain that information (Figures 1.6–1.8). A diagnosis that is accurate is critical to determine presurgical treatment, what type of surgery would be best, and what sort of prognosis a patient can expect [2]. A comparable classification system has been suggested for intramural and subserosal fibroids in order to describe what degree of myometrial involvement exists (see Chapter 2 for the detailed classification system). Three-dimensional ultrasound is becoming an increasingly valuable imaging tool to map out the relationship between the fibroid and the endometrial cavity.

Diagnosis

Two-dimensional ultrasound is the traditional manner of imaging fibroids, although other imaging modalities exist. For ideal visualization of fibroids, especially of their outline, the best technique uses a transvaginal scan (TVS) (see Figures 1.3–1.5). With a transvaginal approach, the ultrasound probe is closer to the uterus, which allows a higher frequency to be used. This higher frequency provides better definition of the tissues. A patient should empty her bladder first before a TVS is done. The TVS transducer is curvilinear, multifrequency, and endocavity, with a central frequency that is usually 6.5 MHz. The ultrasound beam can be highly attenuated by fibroids due to fibroids' dense and mixed tissue composition. Thus, poor through transmission and shadowing may result. As a result of this attenuation, sometimes a lower frequency is used to achieve better penetration of the fibroid in order to see the posterior outline. When a uterus is significantly burdened by fibroids, a TVS can fail to visualize the entire uterus, and a transabdominal ultrasound (TAS) is warranted as well.

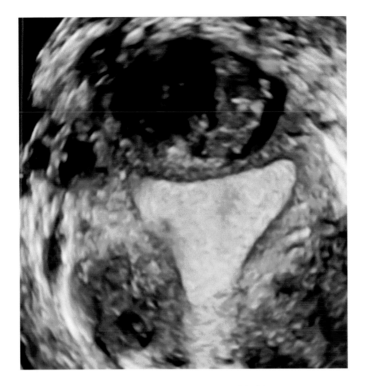

FIGURE 1.6   Three-dimensional ultrasound showing fundal intramural fibroid.

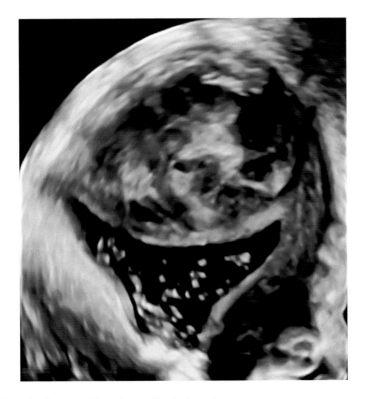

FIGURE 1.7   SIS showing intramural fibroid protruding in the cavity.

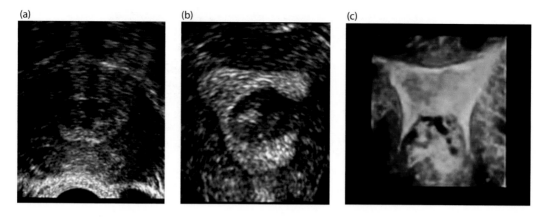

FIGURE 1.8 Submucosal fibroid in three-dimensional (3D) view: (a) transverse section; (b) coronal section; (c) rendered 3D ultrasound.

TAS uses a curvilinear, multihertz abdominal transducer that has a central frequency of 3.5 MHz. The transabdominal approach gives a larger visual perspective to allow for adequate visualization of an enlarged uterus. The abdominal transducer also can use lower frequencies to achieve better penetration of tissue. Additionally, harmonic selection as well as higher power settings can improve the visualization of fibroids on ultrasound. The TAS usually requires a full bladder to see pelvic organs, but such techniques may be unnecessary when the uterus is significantly enlarged with fibroids. This difference is often because the bowel loops that often obscure pelvic organs have been displaced by the large fibroid uterus.

The specific appearance of a fibroid's outline can be well demonstrated on TVS, even of very small fibroids, because of the fibroid's pseudocapsule. The fibroid has a mixed tissue composition such that a heterogenous echo pattern develops on ultrasound. This echo can be highly attenuating for some fibroids. A fibroid should have a definite outline because heterogenous myometrium without a defined margin could be adenomyosis instead. Fibroids are typically hypoechoic when compared to neighboring myometrium, but then sometimes they can be isoechoic (or even hyperechoic if fatty or fibrous changes have occurred). Cystic degeneration of fibroids can be visualized on ultrasound as a central anechoic area that can contain internal echoes or fluid/fluid levels [3] (Figure 1.9). When fibroid tissue has been replaced with fibrous tissue, there is a total increase in reflectivity on ultrasound. Calcification of fibroids can also occur and is seen as echogenic foci or a bright outer rim that causes posterior acoustic shadowing on ultrasound.

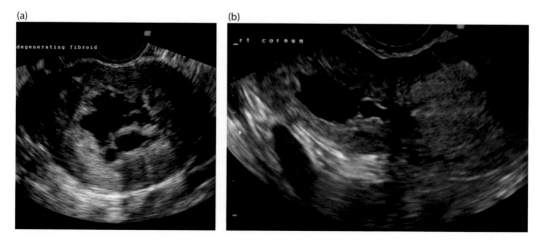

FIGURE 1.9 (a,b) Degenerating fibroids.

(a)

(b)

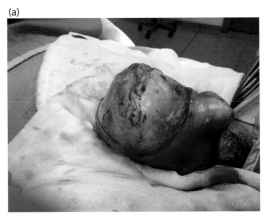 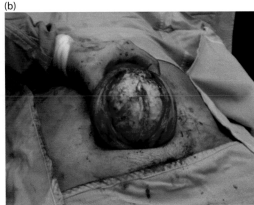

FIGURE 1.10   (a,b) Myomectomy showing removal of intramural fibroid.

Fertility

How fibroids affect fertility is of great importance to reproductive medicine practitioners (see Chapter 3), and many uncertainties remain. Fibroids become symptomatic usually after the age of 35 years, which is the age when fertility starts to decline. However, it is beneficial to first examine how fibroids may affect fertility and then specifically examine the effects of fibroids on *in vitro* fertilization (IVF) outcomes.

Conception

The fact that delayed conception is more frequent in women with fibroids had been highlighted many years ago. In a retrospective study of women with uterine fibroids who presented in labor, 43% of women had at least a 2-year history of infertility [4]. More importantly, the spontaneous conception and live birth rates that follow removal of fibroids (Figure 1.10) may provide indirect evidence that fibroids may have played an important role in impeding pregnancy and contributed to subfertility. In one study, it was reported that the cumulative live birth rate following myomectomy was 50% after 1 year of surgery, with more pregnancies occurring in the second year but at a lower frequency and hardly any beyond 24 months of observation [5] (Figure 1.11). The cumulative chance of pregnancy was obviously affected by age, as reported in another study [6] (Figure 1.12).

Miscarriage

- Many studies looking at the relationship between fibroids and miscarriage examine intramural fibroids, rather than submucosal fibroids [7]. In several studies, intramural fibroids were associated with an increase in miscarriage rate (see Chapter 4) from 8% to 15% [7]. Additionally, multiple fibroids, as opposed to a single fibroid, are a significant risk factor for miscarriage [8]. In one review, miscarriage rates dropped from 41% to 19% after myomectomy for patients with symptomatic fibroids [9]. However, a recent study reported that the hazard ratio (HR) for miscarriage is increased in the presence of uterine fibroids (HR = 1.29%, 95% [CI]: 1.02, 1.64), but after adjusting for the confounding variables—maternal age, race/ethnicity, alcohol use, prior termination of pregnancy, and parity—this increased risk disappeared when adjusted (HR = 0.83%, 95% CI: 0.63, 1.08) [10].

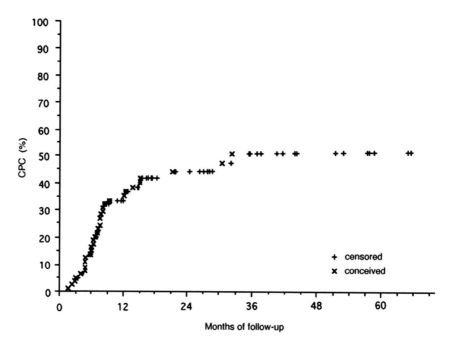

FIGURE 1.11 Cumulative probability of spontaneous intrauterine pregnancy after myomectomy using the Kaplan and Meier method (time 0 is the date of the myomectomy). (From Fauconnier A et al. *Hum Reprod.* 2000;15:1751–7. With permission.)

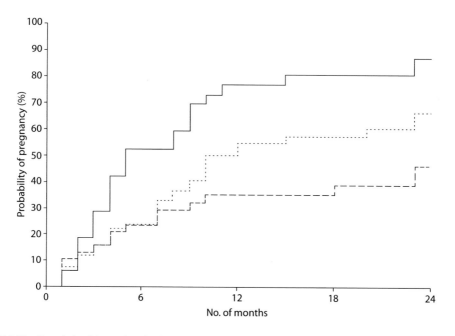

FIGURE 1.12 Cumulative 24-month probability of pregnancy in 138 women who underwent myomectomy, 32 of whom were younger than 30 years of age (-------------), 69 of whom were 30 to 35 years of age (.........), and 38 of whom were older than 35 years of age (- - - - - -) (log rank test, $\chi^2_2 = 12.05$, $P = .0024$). (From Vercellini P et al. *Fertil Steril.* 1999;72:109–14. With permission.)

In Vitro Fertilization Outcome

It is suggested by the literature that the number of women who can attribute their infertility as solely due to fibroids is very low (1%–2.4%) [11]. One study argued that fertility was reduced as a result of fibroids by identifying that 43% of women with fibroids had at least a 2-year history of infertility [12]. Other prospective studies examined how fibroids affect IVF patients and found reduced success in the patients with fibroids [13,14]. Chapter 2 provides further details on the relationship between fibroids and IVF outcomes.

Medical management for fibroids is discussed in Chapter 6, and interventional radiological procedures are discussed in Chapter 9. The roles of ultrasound and MRI before surgery are discussed in Chapters 7 and 8. Removal of submucosal fibroids is the gold standard for improving fertility (see Chapter 10). For intramural fibroids, however, the value of removing the fibroid is more controversial, especially when the cavity is not deformed by the fibroid. One study found significantly lower implantation rates, clinical pregnancy rates, and live birth rates in women with intramural fibroids undergoing IVF as compared to a control group [15]. However, the evidence is conflicted on the impact of fibroid size, number, type, and extent of symptoms [16]. That stated, some studies demonstrate an increased spontaneous conception rate after myomectomy of 50% to 60% [12], with decreased rates of first- and second-trimester miscarriages [9,17].

Thus, while a general consensus exists in the literature that fibroids do affect fertility, what to do with that information is still unknown. It has not been established that removal of fibroids before attempting IVF could impact the outcome [18–25]. Unfortunately, because no randomized controlled trials have addressed the value of myomectomy, and methodological limitations of the literature exist, no obvious guidelines for the management of fibroids in IVF patients have been established. For these reasons, surgical treatment of fibroids before IVF is an individualized decision that considers fibroid symptoms, reproductive history (including any previous failed IVF attempts), and patient preference (see Chapters 2 and 11).

REFERENCES

1. Practice Committee of the ASRM. Myomas and reproductive function. *Fertil Steril.* 2004;82:5111–16.
2. Wamsteker K, and de Blok S. Resection of intrauterine fibroids. In: Lewis BV, and Magos AL (eds). *Endometrial Ablation.* Edinburgh, UK: Churchill Livingstone, 1993.
3. Reddy N, Jain KA, and Gerscovich EO. A degenerating cystic uterine fibroid mimicking an endometrioma on sonography. *J Ultrasound Med.* 2003;22(9):973–6.
4. Hasan F, Arumıgam K, and Sivanesaratnam V. Uterine leiomyomata in pregnancy. *Int J Gynecol Obstet.* 1990;34:45–8.
5. Fauconnier A, Dubuisson JB, Ancel PY et al. Prognostic factors of reproductive outcome after myomectomy in infertile patients. *Hum Reprod.* 2000;15(8):1751–7.
6. Vercellini P, Maddalena S, De Giorgi O et al. Determinants of reproductive outcome after abdominal myomectomy for infertility. *Fertil Steril.* 1999;72(1):109–14.
7. Klatsky P, Tran D, Caughey A, and Fujimoto V. Fibroids and reproductive outcomes: A systematic literature review from conception to delivery. *Am J Obstet Gynecol.* 2008;198(4):357–66.
8. Benson CB, Chow JS, Chang-Lee W et al. Outcome of pregnancies in women with uterine leiomyomas identified by sonography in the first trimester. *J Clin Ultrasound.* 2001;29:261–4.
9. Buttram VC Jr and Reiter RC. Uterine leiomyomata: Etiology, symptomology, and management. *Fertil Steril.* 1981;36:433–45.
10. Hartmann KE, Velez Edwards DR, Savitz DA et al. Prospective cohort study of uterine fibroids and miscarriage risk. *Am J Epidemiol.* 2017;186(10):1140–8.
11. Donnez J and Jadoul P. What are the implications of myomas on fertility? A need for a debate? *Hum Reprod.* 2002;17(6):1424–30.
12. Hasan F, Arumugam K, and Sivanesaratnam V. Uterine leiomyomata in pregnancy. *Int J Gynaecol Obstet.* 1990;34:45–58.

13. Hart R, Khalaf Y, Yeong CT et al. A prospective controlled study of the effect of intramural uterine fibroids on the outcome of assisted conception. *Hum Reprod*. 2001;16:2411–17.

14. Check JH, Choe JK, Lee G, and Dietterich C. The effect on IVF outcome of small intramural fibroids not compressing the uterine cavity as determined by a prospective matched control study. *Hum Reprod*. 2002;17:1244–8.

15. Bai X, Lin Y, Chen Y, and Ma C. The impact of FIGO type 3 fibroids on in-vitro fertilization outcomes: A nested retrospective case-control study. *Eur J Obstet Gynecol Reprod Biol*. 2020;247:176–80.

16. Pritts EA. Fibroids and infertility: A systematic review. *Obstet Gynecol Surv*. 2001;56:483–91.

17. Bulletti C, De Zeigler D, Setti P et al. Myomas, pregnancy outcome and *in vitro* fertilization. *Ann NY Acad Sci*. 2004;1034:84–92.

18. Farhi J, Ashkenazi J, Feldberg D et al. The effects of uterine leiomyomata on in-vitro fertilization treatment. *Hum Reprod*. 1995;10:2576–8.

19. Elder-Geva T, Meagher S, Healy DL et al. Effect of intramural subserosal, and submucosal uterine fibroids on the outcome of assisted reproductive technology treatment. *Fertil Steril*. 1998;70:687–91.

20. Shokeir TA. Hysteroscopic management in submucous fibroids to improve fertility. *Arch Gynecol Obstet*. 2005;273(1):50–4.

21. Narayan R and Rajat Goswamy K. Treatment of submucous fibroids, and outcome of assisted conception. *J Am Assoc Gynecol Laparosc*. 1994;1:307–11.

22. Stovall DW, Parrish SB, Van Voorhis BJ et al. Uterine leiomyomas reduce the efficacy of reproduction cycles. *Hum Reprod*. 1998;13:192–7.

23. Rinehart J. Myomas and infertility: Small intramural myomas do not reduce pregnancy rate *in vitro* fertilization. *Presented at the 53rd annual meeting of the American Society for Reproductive Medicine*, Cincinnati, Ohio, 1997;18–22.

24. Yarali H and Bukulmez O. The effect of intramural and subserous uterine fibroids on implantation and clinical pregnancy rates in patients having intracytoplasmic sperm injection. *Arch Gynecol Obstet*. 2002;266:30–3.

25. Surrey ES, Leitz AK, and Schoolcraft WB. Impact of intramural leiomyomata in patients with a normal endometrial cavity on *in vitro* fertilization-embryo transfer cycle outcome. *Fertil Steril*. 2001;75:405–10.

2

Fibroids and Assisted Reproduction Technology

Eman A. Elgindy

CONTENTS

Introduction

Fibroids are the most common benign gynecological tumors, affecting 20%–50% of women [1]. They are among the factors that may adversely affect embryo implantation and assisted reproduction technology (ART) outcomes. The current chapter explores the evidence regarding the impact of different fibroid types on ART outcome with stratification of their impact based on the fibroid characteristics. The available treatment options that are used to try to improve ART outcome in these patients is highlighted in accordance with the latest published evidence. This would include surgical, medical, and radiological interventions.

Risk Factors

The risk factors for fibroids are demonstrated in Figure 2.1 [2]. Age and race are known risk factors for the development of fibroids. Black women have more than a threefold increase in the prevalence of uterine fibroid than white women [3]. Moreover, fibroid growth rate has been linked with race, as women of African origin have a relatively constant rate throughout their reproductive life, whereas in

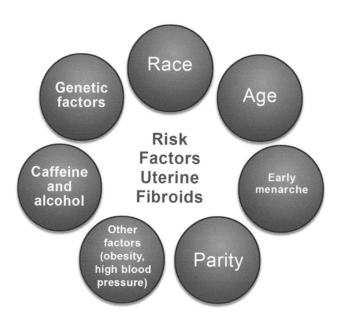

FIGURE 2.1   Risk factors for fibroids. Race, age, early menarche, nulliparity, obesity, hypertension, caffeine and alcohol abuse, as well as genetic alterations are included. (Reproduced with Open Access from Donnez J and Dolmans MM. *Hum Reprod Update*. 2016;22[6]:665–86.)

Caucasian women, myomas have a faster growth rate until the age of 35 years and a slower rate after 45 years [4]. Additionally, other factors, such as early menarche, nulliparity, obesity, polycystic ovary syndrome, hypertension, and diabetes, as well as caffeine and alcohol consumption, have been found, in some studies, to be associated with an increased risk of developing fibroids [5,6].

Chromosomal defects, genetics, epigenetic alterations, steroid hormones, cytokines, chemokines, and growth factors are all hypothesized to have important roles in the initiation and development of this tumor [7–13]. Estrogens were believed initially to be responsible for fibroid growth and differentiation. However, progesterone and its receptors (PR-A and PR-B) are now believed to have a pivotal role in the growth, differentiation, and proliferation of myomas [14,15].

Classification

Fibroids can be subserosal, intramural (IM), or submucosal (SM) in location (see Figures 1.1, 1.3–1.5). However, the FIGO classification, introduced in 2011 by the International Federation of Gynecology and Obstetrics, has been based on the relationship of the myoma with the uterine wall [16]. Eight types of myomas have been described as well as a hybrid class (association of two types of myomas) (Figure 2.2) [2]. For a certain category of fibroids, two numbers may be given (e.g., 2–5), the first one referring to the relationship with the endometrium and the second one with the serosa. This type can indirectly indicate the size of fibroid, which extends throughout the uterine wall, protruding into the cavity and at the same time distorting the outline of the uterus (types 2–5).

Fibroid and Assisted Reproduction Technology Outcomes: Current Evidence

ART has evolved as an established modality to treat infertile couples and is employed for almost all types of infertility. Despite advances in ART, the change of embryo implantation is still considered relatively low. Uterine fibroid is among the factors that may adversely affect implantation and ART outcomes [17]. A study including patients who had *in vitro* fertilization (IVF)/intracytoplasmic sperm injection

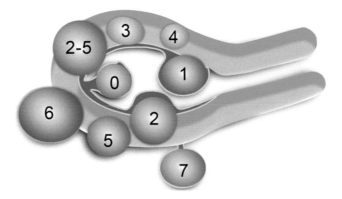

FIGURE 2.2 FIGO classification of fibroids according to Munro et al. (2011). Types are from 0 to 8. 0 = Intracavitary pedunculated; 1 = submucosal, greater than 50% intracavitary; 2 = submucosal, less than 50% intracavitary; 3 = 100% intramural, contacting with the endometrium; 4 = intramural; 5 = subserosal intramural; 6 = subserosal, less than 50% intramural; 7 = pedunculated subserosal; 8 = others (like cervical and parasitic). Two numbers can be given (e.g., 2–5), the first refers to the fibroid relation with endometrium, and the second refers to its relation with serosa. (Reproduced with Open Access from Donnez J and Dolmans MM. *Hum Reprod Update*. 2016;22[6]:665–86.)

(ICSI) reported an incidence of 26.7% for uterine fibroids [18]. The possible adverse effect of fibroid on ART outcome might be explained by the alteration in uterine vascular perfusion, endometrial function, myometrial contractility, gamete migration, myometrial/endometrial gene expression, as well as in vital markers for endometrial receptivity [19–23]. However, the impact of fibroid on ART appears to depend on its type, size, and number.

Subserosal Fibroids

Subserosal myomas do not seem to affect fertility or ART outcome. A systematic review and meta-analysis including 23 studies reported that women with fibroids, irrespective of their location, had significantly lower implantation, clinical pregnancy rate (CPR), and ongoing pregnancy rate (OPR)/live birth rate (LBR) than control subjects. When the analysis was restricted to subserosal fibroids, no difference was observed for any of these outcomes. Therefore, the removal of this fibroid type does not offer any benefit [22]. Infrequently, large subserosal fibroids may impede access to the ovaries for transvaginal ovum pickup and therefore may warrant treatment.

Intramural Fibroids

The impact of IM myomas on infertility and ART outcome has been controversial. Initially, it was believed that myomas not protruding into the intrauterine cavity have no adverse effect on fertility or ART outcome. In 2001, in a systematic review of the evidence, there was no adverse impact of IM fibroids on pregnancy outcome [24]. However, neither the size nor the number of the myomas were taken into consideration. In 2005, Benecke and colleagues in a structured literature review reported contradictory results. They emphasized the presence of a negative impact of IM fibroids on implantation rate and LBR in women undergoing ART. The included studies did not specify a certain cutoff for the size of IM myoma that could affect the outcome [25].

Somigliana et al. (2007) performed an updated meta-analysis, including 16 studies, investigating the influence of fibroids located at different sites in ART cycles. In this critical analysis, the presence of IM myomas was associated with a significantly lower CPR and delivery rate [26]. Additionally, Pritts and colleagues (2009), in their meta-analysis, reported an increased spontaneous abortion rate, decreased implantation rate, and lower ongoing pregnancy/LBRs in the presence of IM fibroids, even with no cavitary involvement [22].

Subsequently, Sunkara and colleagues (2010), in a systematic review and meta-analysis of 19 observational studies, focused on the effect of IM myomas without uterine cavity involvement on ART outcomes. The presence of fibroids was found to reduce both the CPR (by 15%) and the LBR (by 21%) per IVF cycle compared with no fibroids [27].

Several studies have tried to reach a certain cutoff for the size of IM fibroid, above which this fibroid is detrimental to ART outcome. Variable cutoffs, from 2 up to 7 cm, have been suggested in the literature so far, yielding conflicting results [28–31]. There is general agreement, however, that the cutoff for IM fibroids is 4 cm, above which this fibroid is detrimental to ART outcome even without cavity distortion [31].

It is important to point out that the reduction in IVF live births in these non-cavity-distorting IM fibroids does not necessarily mean that their removal will restore the LBRs to the level expected in cases without myomas [27]. A very important clinical dilemma remains unresolved. However, Benecke et al. (2005), in their meta-analysis, suggested that the removal of IM fibroid, at least in cases with previously failed IVF cycles, might improve the outcome. They, however, emphasized the importance of performing further studies before suggesting such recommendations [25].

Pritts et al. (2009), in their meta-analysis, emphasized the absence of clear evidence that myomectomy for these lesions will improve the outcome. They recommended performing high-quality studies to detect the value of myomectomy for IM fibroids, with emphasis on issues such as size, number, and proximity to the endometrium [22]. Further, Sunkara and colleagues (2010) highlighted that routine myomectomy for these women is not yet justified, and there is a need to perform a risk-benefit analysis for this surgical intervention [27].

A prospective, controlled study was performed to evaluate whether fibroid removal prior to conception may improve pregnancy rates and pregnancy maintenance. Women with IM fibroids and trying to conceive for at least 1 year without success were included. After myomectomy, pregnancy rates were 56.5% in cases of IM and 35.5% in cases of IM-subserosal fibroids, respectively. For patients with fibroid who did not undergo surgery, CPRs were 41% in women with IM and 21.43% in women with IM-subserosal fibroids. The results were not statistically significant; however, the investigators suggested a possible beneficial role for removing IM fibroids. This study, however, was in non-ART cycles [32].

In an interesting study, the cost-effectiveness of myomectomy followed by ART or ART with IM myoma(s) *in situ* was analyzed. A decision tree mathematical model was used with sensitivity analysis analyzing published data of eight articles as inputs for costs and probabilities. Pre-ART IM myomectomy was cost effective when the OPR in the presence of *in situ* myomas was less than 15.4%. Meanwhile, when the OPR was 15.4% or greater in the presence of myoma, myomectomy was reported to be cost effective only if pregnancy increased by at least 9.6% [33].

Submucosal Fibroids

Regarding SM fibroids, the literature is relatively less uncertain. Current evidence underscores their potential detrimental effect on fertility and ART outcome. Pregnancy and implantation rates are significantly lower in patients with SM fibroids. Surgical treatment should be considered in these patients before resorting to ART treatment [22,34].

In the meta-analysis and systematic review by Pritts et al. (2009), women with SM fibroids had a significantly lower CPR, implantation rate, and OPR/LBR, and a significantly higher spontaneous miscarriage rate compared with infertile women without fibroids. Importantly, the CPR was indeed higher after performing myomectomy in the SM fibroid group (relative risk = 2.034%, 95% confidence interval = 1.081–3.826, $P = .02$) [22].

Treatment of Fibroids from the Fertility Aspect

Myomectomy is the standard treatment for SM and IM fibroids before ART. Minimally invasive approaches such as hysteroscopy and laparoscopy have gained in popularity over the past several years.

Meanwhile, semi-invasive approaches employing imaging and medical treatment have been introduced in the updated management of these lesions.

Surgical Treatment

Surgery for Submucosal Fibroids

Hysteroscopy is the optimal approach to deal with most SM fibroids. The use of mechanical instruments (scissors and mechanical "cold" loops), electrocautery (vaporizing electrodes and thermal loops), laser fibers ("touch" and "nontouch" technique) [35,36], and/or morcellation [37] have been described. The use of resectoscope with electrical energy is the most widely applied technique [37]. There is, however, concern from the use of monopolar diathermy and its likely damaging effect on the surrounding healthy myometrium and endometrium, mainly in type 1 or 2 FIGO classification fibroid, with possible poorly defined cleavage plane [37,38]. The use of bipolar instruments was suggested to be much safer, as the current will only pass through the tissue with which the thermal instrument comes into contact, thus minimizing injury to adjacent structures [37]. Additionally, the concept of "cold loop" myomectomy has been introduced. This combines both monopolar electrocautery for excising the intracavitary component and mechanical blunt dissection for enucleating the IM part of the fibroid [37,39].

Large sessile SM myomas may require a two-step procedure. During the first step, resection of the protruding portion of the myoma occurs. Interestingly, myometrial thickness was shown to increase upon removing myoma slices during surgery [40]. This leads to protrusion of the remaining IM portion into the uterine cavity. During the second-step hysteroscopy, complete resection of the residual IM part, which has largely moved toward the intrauterine cavity, can be accomplished easily.

Surgery for Intramural Fibroids

Laparoscopy, open abdominal surgery, or a combination of both modalities (laparoscopic-assisted myomectomy) can be performed for IM fibroids.

Laparoscopy appears advantageous with less severe postoperative morbidity and faster recovery [41]. The selection of surgical approach should be individualized according to the size, number, and location of fibroids as well as the surgeon's skill [42]. Laparoscopic myomectomy may not be feasible in the presence of an IM fibroid greater than 10–12 cm and/or multiple fibroids (four or more) in different sites of the uterus, which necessities numerous incisions [2,43].

In a Cochrane Systematic Review, open versus laparoscopic myomectomy was compared in two studies. There was no significant effect of the used modality on LBR, ongoing CPR, pregnancy rate, miscarriage rate, preterm labor rate, and cesarean section rate [44].

Alternatives to Surgical Interference

Uterine Artery Embolization

In uterine artery embolization (UAE), ischemic necrosis of the fibroid is targeted with subsequent marked decline in fibroid volume. A decreased uterine volume up to 50% and improvement of symptoms were reported in some studies [45].

However, fertility after UAE has been questioned, and the impact of this procedure on ovarian reserve is a considerable concern. In initial reports, transient or permanent amenorrhea and symptoms of ovarian failure were reported in up to 5% of women who underwent UAE [46]. In a randomized controlled trial (RCT) comparing UAE and myomectomy, the UAE procedure was associated with less pregnancies and more miscarriages than myomectomy [47]. Further, 66 women who underwent UAE were prospectively followed for almost 3 years, and 31 of these cases were seeking pregnancy. Only 1 of these 31 achieved pregnancy [48]. Zupi et al. (2016) highlighted the results and complications of the UAE procedure. They underscored that the desire for future pregnancy is a relative contraindication for this procedure, as the available data in the literature cannot ensure a good fertility potential [49].

Focused Ultrasound Treatment

This is a noninvasive modality to treat uterine myoma. The high-intensity, focused ultrasound energy is directed to the fibroid with subsequent coagulation tissue necrosis of the fibroid without damaging nearby tissues. This treatment is guided with the use of magnetic resonance (high-frequency magnetic resonance–guided focused ultrasound surgery [MRgFUS]) or ultrasound (ultrasound-guided high-intensity focused ultrasound [USgHIFU]).

Although the damage to surrounding tissue is expected to be minimal, possible detrimental effects on critical neighboring structures cannot be excluded [50].

Clark et al. (2014), in their systematic review, emphasized that hypointense fibroids were associated with increased treatment success, in comparison to hyperintense ones. Notably, hyperintense fibroids were present in about 59% of young women. Major limitations to this modality are as follows: (1) this technique does not apply to all patients, (2) financial burden, and (3) fertility potential needs further study [51].

The available data in literature are not enough. Approximately 30% of women underwent further fibroid surgery or procedures 2 years after MRgFUS [52]. Currently, there is upgrading for screening, and valid magnetic resonance imaging (MRI)-based prediction models are being advanced for assessing the therapeutic responses and decreasing treatment failure [53]. Regarding ovarian reserve, in a recent study, anti-müllerian hormone (AMH) levels before and 6 months after high-intensity focused ultrasound (HIFU) ablation were measured in 79 cases. No significant difference in AMH levels existed between the two time points [54]. However, follow-up of ovarian reserve and pregnancy outcome are warranted in large-scale prospective studies.

Medical Treatment

Medical management of fibroids exploits the progesterone and estrogen responsiveness of uterine fibroids. Medical treatment, however, is not curative for fibroids. It has been considered as an option for symptom control and fibroid volume reduction. GnRH analogs have been commonly used. Other therapies including aromatase inhibitors, selective estrogen receptor modulators, and selective progesterone receptor modulators (SPRMs) have also been tried without the hypoestrogenic effects of the GnRH analogs. Currently, the two most studied and promising medical treatments are the GnRH agonist and SPRMs [2].

GnRH Agonists

GnRH agonists induce a state of hypoestrogenemia and temporary menopause with subsequent shrinkage of fibroids [55]. They cannot be used for long periods due to their side effects, including bone loss and hot flushes.

In patients with large SM fibroids, the use of a preoperative agonist has the following advantages: (1) correction of anemia, (2) decrease of myoma size, (3) reduction in endometrial thickness and vascularization with enhanced visibility and decrease in fluid absorption, and (4) the option of scheduling operative hysteroscopy at any time [55,56]. However, agonists are not recommended for routine use in SM fibroids due to increased cost, side effects, as well as postinjection endometrial bleeding due to the flare-up effect [37].

Regarding laparoscopic and/or abdominal myomectomy, it was suggested that using a preoperative agonist might obscure the cleavage plane between the pseudocapsule and healthy myometrium. Concerns from extensive dissection of the fibroid, distortion of the pseudocapsule, and increased operative time were reported [57]. However, in a systematic review and meta-analysis, the use of an agonist prior to laparotomic and laparoscopic myomectomy had decreased intraoperative blood loss and the frequency of blood transfusions. Enucleation time for myoma and difficulty of surgery did not significantly increase with use of agonist pretreatment [58].

Lethaby et al. (2017), in a recent Cochrane review, underscored the presence of clear evidence that use of a preoperative agonist reduces fibroid volume and increases preoperative hemoglobin levels; however, it does increase the incidence of hot flushes [59].

Selective Progesterone Receptor Modulators

The crucial role of progesterone in the development and growth of myomas has been established. Therefore, the progesterone pathway can be modulated using SPRMs [60–62]. These compounds exert either an agonistic or antagonistic effect on progesterone receptors. The mechanism of action of SPRMs on the receptors depends on their structure and how they alter the receptor conformation, which will dictate whether SPRM will act more as an agonist or antagonist [63].

Four family members of SPRMs have been investigated in clinical trials: mifepristone, asoprisnil, ulipristal acetate (UPA), and telapristone acetate [60–62]. The two most studied drugs have been mifepristone and UPA. Some studies reported a significant reduction of myoma size and improvement in symptoms upon using mifepristone [64,65]. However, a Cochrane review found no clear evidence for this. Mifepristone reduced heavy menstrual bleeding and improved quality of life, but it did not significantly reduce fibroid volume [66].

Meanwhile, encouraging results have been shown with the latest SPRM, UPA, in terms of safety and efficacy. UPA was compared to GnRH agonist (leuprolide acetate) and placebo in two RCTs. There was more control of uterine bleeding in more than 90% of cases receiving 3 months of UPA, and the time to bleeding control was longer in the GnRH agonist group (21 days) than in the UPA group (5–7 days). More sustained effect was observed with the UPA group (up to 6 months); meanwhile, rapid regrowth of the fibroid occurred in the agonist group who did not undergo surgery after the 3 months of treatment [67,68].

In a recent Cochrane review, there was a more significant decrease in uterine volume when using the agonist than when using the UPA (−47% with agonist compared to −20% and −22% with 5 mg and 10 mg UPA). Control of uterine bleeding and hemoglobin levels was comparable between agonist and UPA. Significant hot flushes developed with the agonist use [59].

In another recent Cochrane review, there was no difference between leuprolide acetate and UPA regarding bleeding symptoms and improved quality of life. The investigators emphasized that evidence is currently insufficient to show different levels of effectiveness between UPA and leuprolide [69].

See Chapter 6 for further details.

Algorithms for Fibroid Management

There is no doubt that surgery is indicated in certain fibroid cases before ART. We need to establish a systematic approach to these cases and try to accomplish less invasive surgery even with the use of endoscopy. The site of fibroids according to FIGO classification [16], the number, and myoma volume are important determinant factors [42].

Type 0 Myomas

Hysteroscopic myomectomy is the ultimate approach [2].

Type 1 and 2 Myomas

The strategy for these myomas depends on the size, presence of anemia, and surgeon skill. Hysteroscopic myomectomy is a relatively straightforward procedure for experienced surgeons in the case of type 1 myoma, less than 3 cm, in the absence of anemia. However, pre-hysteroscopic medical treatment (GnRH agonist or UTA) can be applied in cases of type 1 myoma larger than 3 cm, in cases with type 2, and in patients with type 1 or 2 presenting with anemia. This may induce fibroid shrinkage and enable an easier approach in the presence of a better general condition [2,70].

It was reported that type 2 myoma might significantly regress in some cases, so that they no longer disturb the endometrial cavity, and their size becomes lower than the reported detrimental cutoff size;

therefore, surgery can be avoided [71]. However, this needs to be tested in large-scale studies. Importantly, it has been suggested that large (greater than 3 cm), type 2 SM fibroids occupying the entire myometrium are better managed through laparoscopy [72]. Importantly, surgeon skill and preference are major determinants in dealing with type 2 myomas.

Types 3 through 5 Myomas (Single or Multiple)

Laparoscopic and/or abdominal myomectomy are the standard procedure. Laparoscopic myomectomy is initially recommended. However, the decision depends on the size, number, and surgeon skill, as mentioned earlier in this chapter.

If myomas are multiple (two or more), large, or of different types, preoperative medical treatment (agonist or UPA) may be considered [59,71].

In general, one course of 3 months' treatment is tried. Two courses of 3 months' treatment with UPA were recommended in cases of large, multiple (two or more), or different types of myomas [2,71]. Significant myoma regression was reported in some cases (greater than 50% decrease in volume), so that the endometrial cavity was not distorted, and patients had undergone ART without surgery [2]. In a recent Cochrane review, it was emphasized that replication of these studies is recommended before making firm conclusions. Future studies should target cost-effectiveness and identify the group of fibroid patients who would benefit from this approach [59].

Conclusion

Fibroids are common in women of reproductive age. Their presence could adversely affect natural fertility and ART outcomes. Existing evidence indicates that SM and IM fibroids, even without uterine cavity involvement, may have a detrimental effect on ART outcome. Removal of SM fibroids appears to improve reproductive outcome. There is, however, insufficient evidence that removing IM fibroids would result in a favorable impact on ART outcome.

The size, number, location, as well as surgeon's experience and available equipment are important determinants in choosing the appropriate therapeutic approach. In women who are desirous of pregnancy, surgery is the recommended modality, using endoscopy whenever possible. Nonsurgical therapeutic approaches, such as UAE, MRgFUS, and USgHIFU may be considered when surgery is not feasible or deemed too risky. There are, however, insufficient data in the literature to ensure a good fertility potential.

Medical treatment, though it has its place, is mainly for preoperative preparation and for only a limited period of time.

REFERENCES

1. Baird DD, Dunson DB, Hill MC et al. High cumulative incidence of uterine leiomyoma in black and white women: Ultrasound evidence. *Am J Obstet Gynecol.* 2003;188:100–7.
2. Donnez J and Dolmans MM. Uterine fibroid management: From the present to the future. *Hum Reprod Update.* 2016;22(6):665–86.
3. Marshall LM, Spiegelman D, Barbieri RL et al. Variation in the incidence of uterine leiomyoma among premenopausal women by age and race. *Obstet Gynecol.* 1997;90:967–73.
4. Peddada SD, Laughlin ShK, Miner K et al. Growth of uterine leiomyomata among premenopausal black and white women. *Proc Natl Acad Sci USA.* 2008;105:19887–92.
5. Wise LA, Palmer JR, Harlow BL et al. Risk of uterine leiomyomata in relation to tobacco, alcohol and caffeine consumption in the Black Women's Health Study. *Hum Reprod.* 2004;19:1746–54.
6. Okolo S. Incidence, aetiology and epidemiology of uterine fibroids. *Best Pract Res Clin Obstet Gynaecol.* 2008;22:571–88.
7. Sandberg AA. Updates on the cytogenetics and molecular genetics of bone and soft tissue tumors: Leiomyoma. *Cancer Genet Cytogenet.* 2005;158:1–26.

8. El-Gharib MN and Elsobky ES. Cytogenetic aberrations and the development of uterine leiomyomata. *J Obstet Gynaecol Res.* 2010;36:101–7.
9. Cha PC, Takahashi A, Hosono N et al. A genome-wide association study identifies three loci associated with susceptibility to uterine fibroids. *Nat Genet.* 2011;43:447–50.
10. Elagaleti GV, Tonk VS, Hakim NM et al. Fusion of HMGA2 to COG5 in uterine leiomyoma. *Cancer Genet Cytogenet.* 2011;202:11–6.
11. Wang T, Zhang X, Obijuru L et al. A micro-RNA signature associated with race, tumor size, and target gene activity in human uterine leiomyomas. *Genes Chromosomes Cancer.* 2007;46:336–47.
12. Navarro A, Yin P, Monsivais D et al. Genome-wide DNA methylation indicates silencing of tumor suppressor genes in uterine leiomyoma. *PLOS ONE.* 2012;7:e33284.
13. Greathouse KL, Bredfeldt T, Everitt JI et al. Environmental estrogens differentially engage the histone methyltransferase EZH2 to increase risk of uterine tumorigenesis. *Mol Cancer Res.* 2012;10:546–57.
14. Kim JJ and Sefton EC. The role of progesterone signaling in the pathogenesis of uterine leiomyoma. *Mol Cell Endocrinol.* 2012;358:223–31.
15. Islam MS, Protic O, Stortoni P et al. Complex networks of multiple factors in the pathogenesis of uterine leiomyoma. *Fertil Steril.* 2013;100:178–93.
16. Munro MG, Critchley HOD, Broder MS et al. FIGO classification system (PALM-COEIN) for causes of abnormal uterine bleeding in nongravid women of reproductive age. *Int J Gynecol Obstet.* 2011;113:3–13.
17. The Practice Committee of the American Society for Reproductive Medicine in collaboration with the Society of Reproductive Surgeons. Myomas and reproductive function. *Fertil Steril.* 2008;90:S125–30.
18. Hart R, Khalaf Y, Yeong CT et al. A prospective controlled study of the effect of intramural uterine fibroids on the outcome of assisted conception. *Hum Reprod.* 2001;11:2411–7.
19. Arslan AA, Gold LI, Mittal K et al. Gene expression studies provide clues to the pathogenesis of uterine leiomyoma: New evidence and a systematic review. *Hum Reprod.* 2005;20:852–63.
20. Ng EH, Chan CC, and Tang OS. Endometrial and subendometrial blood flow measured by three-dimensional power Doppler ultrasound in patients with small intramural uterine fibroids during IVF treatment. *Hum Reprod.* 2005;20:501–6.
21. Nishino M, Togashi K, Nakai A et al. Uterine contractions evaluated on cine MR imaging in patients with uterine leiomyomas. *Eur J Radiol.* 2005;53:142–6.
22. Pritts EA, Parker WH, and Olive DL. Fibroids and infertility: An updated systematic review of the evidence. *Fertil Steril.* 2009;91:1215–23.
23. Taylor HS. Fibroids: When should they be removed to improve *in vitro* fertilization success? *Fertil Steril.* 2018;109:784–5.
24. Pritts EA. Fibroids and infertility: A systematic review of the evidence. *Obstet Gynecol Survey.* 2001;56:483–91.
25. Benecke C, Kruger TF, Siebert TI et al. Effect of fibroids on fertility in patients undergoing assisted reproduction, a structured literature review. *Gynecol Obstet Invest.* 2005;59:225–30.
26. Somigliana E, Vercellini P, Daguati R et al. Fibroids and female reproduction: A critical analysis of the evidence. *Hum Reprod Update.* 2007;13:465–76.
27. Sunkara SK, Khairy M, El-Toukhy T et al. The effect of intramural fibroids without uterine cavity involvement on the outcome of IVF treatment: A systematic review and meta-analysis. *Hum Reprod.* 2010;25:418–29.
28. Yan L, Ding L, Li C et al. Effect of fibroids not distorting the endometrial cavity on the outcome of *in vitro* fertilization treatment: A retrospective cohort study. *Fertil Steril.* 2014;101:716–21.
29. Yan L, Yuq Zang Y, Guo Z et al. Effect of type 3 intramural fibroids on endometrial fertilization—Intracytoplasmic sperm injection outcomes as: A retrospective cohort study. *Fertil Steril.* 2018;109:817–22.
30. Jun SH, Ginsburg ES, Racowsky C et al. Uterine leiomyomas and their effect on *in vitro* fertilization outcome: A retrospective study. *J Assist Reprod Genetics.* 2001;18:139–43.
31. Zepiridis LI, Grimbizis GF, and Tarlatsis BC. Infertility and uterine fibroids. *Best Pract Res Clin Obstet Gynaecol.* 2016;34:66–73.
32. Casini ML, Rossi F, Agostini R et al. Effects of the position of fibroids on fertility. *Gynecol Endocrinol.* 2006;22(2):106–9.
33. Ojo-Carons M, Mumford SL, Armstrong AY et al. Is myomectomy prior to assisted reproductive technology cost effective in women with intramural fibroids? *Gynecol Obstet Invest.* 2016;81(5):442–6.

34. Eldar-Geva T, Meagher S, Healy DL et al. Effect of intramural, subserosal, and submucosal uterine fibroids on the outcome of assisted reproductive technology treatment. *Fertil Steril.* 1998;70(4):687–91.
35. Goldrath MH, Fuller TA, and Segal S. Laser photovaporization of endometrium for the treatment of menorrhagia. *Am J Obstet Gynecol.* 1981;140:14–9.
36. Loffer FD. Hysteroscopic endometrial ablation with the Nd:Yag laser using a nontouch technique. *Obstet Gynecol.* 1987;69:679–82.
37. Sardo ADS, Mazzon I, Bramante S et al. Hysteroscopic myomectomy: A comprehensive review of surgical techniques. *Hum Reprod Update.* 2008;14:101–19.
38. Haimovich S, Eliseeva M, Ospan A et al. Hysteroscopic myomectomy. In: Tinelli A and Malvasi A (eds) *Uterine Myoma, Myomectomy and Minimally Invasive Treatments.* Switzerland: Springer Nature, 2015, pp. 129–51.
39. Mazzon I, Favilli A, Villani V et al. Hysteroscopic myomectomy respecting the pseudocapsule: The cold loop hysteroscopic myomectomy. In: Tinelli A, Pacheco LA and Haimovich S (eds) *Hysteroscopy.* Cham, Switzerland: Springer International, 2018, pp. 363–74.
40. Casadio P, Youssef AM, Spagnolo E et al. Should the myometrial free margin still be considered a limiting factor for hysteroscopic resection of submucous fibroids? A possible answer to an old question. *Fertil Steril.* 2011;95(5):1764–8.
41. Legendre G, Brun JL, and Fernandez H. The place of myomectomy in woman of reproductive age. *J Gynecol Obstet Biol Reprod.* 2011;40:875–84.
42. Carranza-Mamane B, Havelock SQC, Hemmings VBC et al. The management of uterine fibroids in women with otherwise unexplained infertility. *J Obstet Gynaecol Can.* 2015;37(3):277–85.
43. Malzoni M, Tinelli R, Cosentino F et al. Laparoscopy versus minilaparotomy in women with symptomatic uterine myomas: Short-term and fertility results. *Fertil Steril.* 2010; 93(7):2368–73.
44. Metwally M, Cheong YC, and Horne AW. Surgical treatment of fibroids for subfertility. *Cochrane Database Syst Rev* 2012;(11):CD003857.
45. Gupta JK, Sinha A, Lumsden MA et al. Uterine artery embolization for symptomatic uterine fibroids. *Cochrane Database Syst Rev.* 2012;(5):CD005073.
46. Chrisman HB, Saker MB, Ryu RK et al. The impact of uterine fibroid embolization on resumption of menses and ovarian function. *J Vasc Interv Radiol.* 2000;11:699–703.
47. Mara M, Maskova J, Fucikova Z et al. Midterm clinical and first reproductive results of a randomized controlled trial comparing uterine fibroid embolization and myomectomy. *Cardiovasc Intervent Radiol.* 2008;31(1):73–85.
48. Torre A, Paullisson B, Fain V et al. Uterine artery embolization for severe symptomatic fibroids: Effects on fertility and symptoms. *Hum Reprod.* 2014;29:490–501.
49. Zupi E, Centini G, Sabbioni L et al. Nonsurgical alternatives for uterine fibroids. *Best Pract Res Clin Obstet Gynaecol.* 2016;34:122–31.
50. Fischer K, McDannold NJ, Tempany CM et al. Potential of minimally invasive procedures in the treatment of uterine fibroids: A focus on magnetic resonance-guided focused ultrasound therapy. *Int J Womens Health.* 2015;7:901–12.
51. Clark NA, Mumford SL, and Segars JH. Reproductive impact of MRI-guided focused ultrasound surgery for fibroids: A systematic review of the evidence. *Curr Opin Obstet Gynecol.* 2014;26:151–61.
52. Jacoby VL, Kohi MP, Poder L et al. PROMISe trial: A pilot, randomized, placebo–controlled trial of magnetic resonance guided focused ultrasound for uterine fibroids. *Fertil Steril.* 2015;S0015-0282:02090-7.
53. Kim YS, Lim HK, Park MJ et al. Screening magnetic resonance imaging-based prediction model for assessing immediate therapeutic response to magnetic resonance imaging-guided high-intensity focused ultrasound ablation of uterine fibroids. *Invest Radiol.* 2016;51:15–24.
54. Lee JS, Hong GY, Lee KH et al. Changes in anti-müllerian hormone levels as a biomarker for ovarian reserve after ultrasound-guided high-intensity focused ultrasound treatment of adenomyosis and uterine fibroid. *BJOG* 2017;124:18–22.
55. Lethaby A, Vollenhoven B, and Sowter M. Pre-operative GnRH analogue therapy before hysterectomy or myomectomy for uterine fibroids. *Cochrane Database Syst Rev.* 2001;(2):CD000547.
56. Doherty L, Mutlu L, Sinclair D et al. Uterine fibroids: Clinical manifestations and contemporary management. *Reprod Sci.* 2014;21(9):1067–92.

57. De Falco M, Staibano S, Mascolo M et al. Leiomyoma pseudocapsule after pre-surgical treatment with gonadotropin-releasing hormone agonists: Relationship between clinical features and immunohistochemical changes. *Eur J Obstet Gynecol Reprod Biol.* 2009;144:44–7.

58. de Milliano I, Twisk M, Ket JC et al. Pre-treatment with GnRHa or ulipristal acetate prior to laparoscopic and laparotomic myomectomy: A systematic review and meta-analysis. *PLOS ONE.* 2017;12(10):e0186158.

59. Lethaby A, Puscasiu L, and Vollenhoven B. Preoperative medical therapy before surgery for uterine fibroids. *Cochrane Database Syst Rev.* 2017;11:CD000547.

60. Bouchard P, Chabbert-Buffet N, and Fauser BC. Selective progesterone receptor modulators in reproductive medicine: Pharmacology, clinical efficacy and safety. *Fertil Steril.* 2011;96(5):1175–89.

61. Bouchard P. Selective progesterone receptor modulators: A class with multiple actions and applications in reproductive endocrinology, and gynecology. *Gynecol Endocrinol.* 2014;30(10):683–4.

62. Whitaker LH, Williams AR, and Critchley HO. Selective progesterone receptor modulators. *Curr Opin Obstet Gynecol.* 2014;26(4):237–42.

63. Moravek MB, Yin P, Ono M et al. Ovarian steroids, stem cells and uterine leiomyoma: Therapeutic implications. *Hum Reprod Update* 2015;21(1):1–12.

64. Engman M, Granberg S, Williams AR et al. Mifepristone for treatment of uterine leiomyoma. A prospective randomized placebo-controlled trial. *Hum Reprod.* 2009;24:1870–9.

65. Bagaria M, Suneja A, Vaid NB et al. Low-dose mifepristone in treatment of uterine leiomyoma: A randomised double-blind placebo-controlled clinical trial. *Aust N Z J Obstet Gynaecol.* 2009;49(1):77–83.

66. Tristan M, Orozco LJ, Steed A et al. Mifepristone for uterine fibroids. *Cochrane Database Syst Rev.* 2012;(8):CD007687.

67. Donnez J, Tatarchuk TF, Bouchard P et al. Ulipristal acetate versus placebo for fibroid treatment before surgery. *N Engl J Med.* 2012a;366:409–20.

68. Donnez J, Tomaszewski J, Vázquez F et al. Ulipristal acetate versus leuprolide acetate for uterine fibroids. *N Engl J Med.* 2012b;366:421–32.

69. Murji A, Whitaker L, Chow TL et al. Selective progesterone receptor modulators (SPRMs) for uterine fibroids. *Cochrane Database Syst Rev.* 2017;4:CD010770.

70. Mas A, Tarazona M, Carrasco JD et al. Updated approaches for management of uterine fibroids. *Int J Womens Health.* 2017;9:607–17.

71. Donnez J, Arriagada P, Donnez O et al. Current management of myomas: The place of medical therapy with the advent of selective progesterone receptor modulators. *Curr Opin Obstet Gynecol.* 2015;27(6):422–31.

72. Closon F and Tulandi T. Uterine myomata: Organ-preserving surgery. Best practice and research. *Clin Obstet Gynaecol.* 2016;35:30–6.

3

Fibroids and Endometrial Receptivity/ Embryo Implantation

Kamaria C. Cayton Vaught, Maria Facadio Antero, Jacqueline Y. Maher, and Chantel I. Cross

CONTENTS

Introduction

Uterine leiomyomas, or fibroids, are the most common benign tumor of the female reproductive tract affecting up to 70% of Caucasian women and 80% of Black women by their late 40s [1]. Given their high prevalence, fibroids can have a significant effect on fertility outcomes, including implantation, ongoing pregnancy, live birth rate, and spontaneous abortion rate [2].

Approximately one out of every four women undergoing assisted reproductive technologies has fibroids [3–5]. The anatomic location of a fibroid is thought to be a defining characteristic that influences the reproductive potential. The gold standard for addressing fibroid-related infertility is myomectomy, which can increase pregnancy and live birth rates upward of 50%–60% in women without other known causes of infertility [6].

Several hypotheses have been proposed to explain the relationship between fibroids and infertility. One mechanism by which fibroids may reduce fertility is through dysregulation of endometrial receptivity. Endometrial receptivity refers to a defined period in the menstrual cycle where the endometrium allows for embryo attachment and invasion, triggering a series of events that culminate in a successful pregnancy.

In this chapter, we review the mechanisms by which fibroids can impact endometrial receptivity. Key mechanisms discussed include mechanical disruption, disruption of implantation (invasion), alteration of the endometrium's vasculature, increased inflammation, and dysregulation of genes important during the window of implantation.

Implantation

Normal Steps of Implantation

The process of embryo implantation is necessary for the establishment of a pregnancy. It involves embryo apposition, adhesion, and invasion into a receptive endometrium (Figure 3.1). In order for implantation to occur and a pregnancy to be established, embryo viability and endometrial receptivity need to be in synchrony, which normally occurs due to complex communication between both the embryo and the endometrium.

Human embryos enter the uterus at around the fifth day after fertilization. At this stage, the embryo is referred to as a blastocyst and consists of an inner cell mass and an outer trophectoderm layer. The inner cell mass gives rise to the fetus, amnion, and vascular components of the placenta, while the trophectoderm becomes the placenta and the chorion. The embryo then interacts with the endometrial epithelium, which, in a paracrine manner, secretes various cytokines, chemokines, and cell adhesion molecules (CAMs) [7–9]. These signals facilitate apposition and adherence of the embryo to optimal implantation sites in the endometrium.

In humans, the endometrium is most receptive to implantation 8–10 days following ovulation [10]. Embryo implantation during this time frame is associated with an 85% ongoing pregnancy rate, whereas implantation on day 11 is associated with an 11% ongoing pregnancy rate [10]. This optimum time frame of endometrium receptivity is termed the *window of implantation* (WOI).

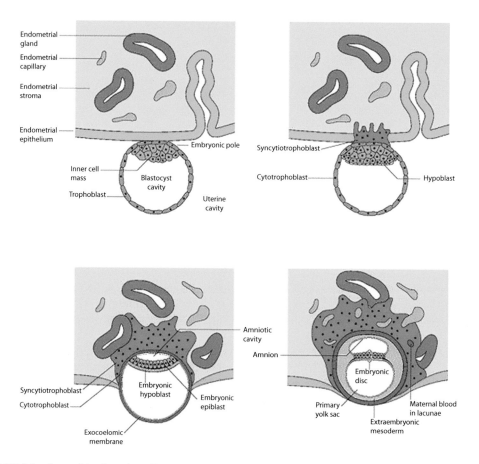

FIGURE 3.1 Steps of implantation. (From Taylor HS, Pal L, Seli E, eds, Conception – Sperm and egg transport, fertilization, implantation and early embryogenesis. In: *Speroff's Clinicl Gynecologic Endocrinology and Infertility*, 9th edn, Wolters Kluwer, Philadelphia, 2020: 174–95. With permission.)

Through the actions of progesterone in the luteal phase, the endometrium becomes thicker and vascular in preparation for implantation. The increase in vascularity and development of stromal spiral arterioles provide a substrate for embryo invasion and implantation. Optimal sites for implantation need to have sufficient depth, vascularity, and nutritional richness to support early placentation. Once the embryo has attached to a receptive area of the endometrium, trophoblast cells invade the maternal circulation to establish the hemochorial placenta. This structure will maintain high blood flow interchange between mother and fetus throughout the pregnancy.

Endometrial Receptivity

As mentioned earlier in this section, timing of embryo implantation is critical as the endometrium is receptive during a very brief window. The endometrium is a dynamic tissue whose growth and regulation are primarily hormone driven, under the control of cyclical estrogen and progesterone exposure. Although histologic criteria for dating the endometrium were established in 1950 as the gold standard for endometrium assessment [11], it turned out to be imperfect secondary to the great intra- and interobserver variability in interpretation and the potential to miss pathologies [12].

Gene transcription regulates histologic and physiologic changes within the endometrium throughout the menstrual cycle. With the advent of the Human Genome Project and the study of different "omics," gene expression profiling became a potential method to investigate endometrial receptivity [13]. Several groups have utilized microarray technology to identify genes within the endometrium and correlate their regulation with specific phases in the menstrual cycle [14–20]. Initial studies looking at RNA transcript analysis and whole genome-wide sequencing were able to identify unique genes that are temporally differentially expressed [19,20]. This allowed the identification of a unique molecular signature for different histologic and physiologic stages of the endometrium during the menstrual cycle.

Several studies have also looked specifically at genes that are regulated during the WOI (Table 3.1) [14–18]. In a review by the Simon group, they further analyzed five independent (and their own) studies of endometrial receptivity genes and identified a consensus of 25 WOI genes between all of the studies that were regulated in the natural cycle [21]. This group went on to be the first to report the sequential molecular development of the WOI in natural cycles, which is the basis of the endometrial receptivity assay (ERA) [22]. The ERA test can determine the specific transcriptomic signature from an endometrial biopsy and identify the WOI in both natural and artificially stimulated cycles [23]. They concluded that there is a well-defined transition from the prereceptive to receptive state of the endometrium and that the WOI is primarily induced by gene activation or a "transcriptional awakening process" rather than gene inactivation [24]. Genes identified that were differentially regulated during the WOI included genes that regulated cell adhesion, suppression of cell proliferation, cell differentiation, proteolysis regulation, up-regulation of metabolism, growth factor, cytokine binding and signaling, immune and inflammatory responses, and responses to wound healing and stress [13].

TABLE 3.1

Studies Comparing Phases of the Menstrual Cycle and Differentially Regulated Genes

Study	Tissues Compared	Biopsy Timing (Prereceptive versus Receptive)	DEG
[16]	LP versus MS	CD 9–11 versus LH + (6–8)	136
[15]	ES versus MS	LH +(2–4) versus LH + (7–9)	693
[14]	LP versus MS	CD 8–10 versus LH + (8–10)	533
[18]	ES versus MS	LH + 3 versus LH + 8	107
[17]	ES versus MS	LH + 2 versus LH + 7	211

Abbreviations: CD, cycle day; DEG, differentially regulated genes; ES, early secretory; LH, luteinizing hormone; LP, late proliferative; MS, midsecretory.

Fibroids and Endometrial Receptivity

Given the high prevalence of fibroids in women of reproductive age, it is not surprising that there is also an association between fibroids and fertility. There are several proposed mechanisms by which fibroids can cause infertility, which range from mechanical effects on gamete transport and implantation, alterations in uterine vasculature, inflammatory effects, and direct impact on gene expression during the WOI. There is a growing body of evidence that supports the concept that fibroids can negatively affect endometrial receptivity through one or more of these mechanisms.

Mechanical Disruptors

Implantation is a highly coordinated process that occurs in a very finite window during the midsecretory phase of the menstrual cycle as previously described in this chapter. At the most rudimentary level, in order for successful implantation to occur, the gametes must be able to travel through the fallopian tubes, and the resulting embryo must travel back to the endometrial cavity. On a macroscopic level, fibroids can directly interfere with implantation by blocking gamete and embryo transport. Fibroids that directly block the lumen of the fallopian tubes can pose as a mechanical barrier to implantation [25].

Gamete transport prior to fertilization is also aided by subtle uterine contractions or uterine peristalsis [26–28]. Uterine peristalsis is bidirectional and primarily moves in an upward direction, from cervix toward the fundus, during the proliferative phase of the endometrium so as to aid sperm transport [28]. The direction of the uterine peristalsis changes during menstruation and proceeds from fundal to cervical [28]. It has been well documented that uterine peristalsis slows and becomes almost undetectable during the luteal phase, especially around the WOI [28,29]. Studies conducted on infertile patients undergoing *in vitro* fertilization (IVF) have found that IVF success rates are reduced in women with high uterine contractility at the time of embryo transfer [30]. A study conducted by Yoshino et al. evaluated the effect of uterine peristalsis and pregnancy rates in infertile women with intramural fibroids [31]. The study group consisted of infertile women with no other obvious cause of infertility other than fibroids (excluding endometriosis) and excluded women with submucosal fibroids. Patients were grouped based on frequency of uterine contractions and found that pregnancy rates were significantly higher in the low-frequency group compared to the high-frequency group (34% in the low-frequency group versus 0% in the high-frequency group, $p < .005$) [31]. A follow-up study by the same author evaluated the effect of myomectomy on subsequent pregnancy rates in patients who were previously assigned to the "high-frequency" group [32]. Fifteen patients were included in the study, and following myomectomy, 14 out of the 15 patients had lower levels of uterine peristalsis and now qualified as "low frequency." The overall pregnancy rate following myomectomy was 40%, and all pregnancies occurred in patients in the low-frequency group [32]. Quiescence of uterine peristalsis appears to be an important mechanical contributor to endometrial receptivity, and intramural fibroids may disrupt this process by promoting increased peristaltic activity. Estrogen appears to promote uterine peristalsis [26,27,32]. Fibroids are known to have an increased expression of the aromatase enzyme, which converts androgens to estrogens [33,34]. Perhaps, the increased aromatase activity in fibroids leads to higher local levels of estrogen, resulting in increased uterine peristalsis and disruption of endometrial receptivity.

Disruption of Implantation

A receptive endometrium is defined by a precise histologic and architectural appearance as well as the up- and downregulation of specific genes, and expression of cytokines and growth factors. The histologic appearance of receptive endometrium is characterized by endometrial glands with abundant stromal edema. The endometrial glands and stroma are essential for implantation. Fibroids appear to be associated with a reduction in the proportion of endometrial glands overlying the fibroids [35]. Moreover, endometrial biopsy specimens that compared the endometrium of women with and without intramural fibroids found that large intramural fibroids are associated with a delay of endometrial development during the WOI [36].

Other components of the uterine architecture are involved in implantation. The junctional zone, which is defined as the innermost myometrial layer, plays a key role in the process of deep placentation of the invading embryo [37]. The myocytes within the junctional zone exhibit differential expression of estrogen and progesterone receptors throughout the menstrual cycle, a feature that is not present in myocytes from the outer myometrial layer [38]. Submucosal fibroids are derived from junctional zone myocytes and thus may negatively impact implantation through disruption of junctional zone function [37,38].

Aside from histoarchitectural alterations in receptivity, specific types of fibroids may differentially impact gene expression profiles of the receptive endometrium. HOXA10 is a transcription factor that is necessary for endometrial receptivity. Mice with a targeted mutation to *Hoxa10* are infertile due to implantation failure [39]. During the midsecretory phase, around the time of implantation, endometrial glands upregulate *HOXA10* expression, whereas stromal expression of *HOXA10* remains constant [39,40]. Submucosal fibroids appear to have a larger impact on *HOXA10* expression when compared to intramural fibroids [40]. Submucosal fibroids are associated with a global reduction in *HOXA10* mRNA expression within the endometrium [40]. Comparatively, the endometria from patients with intramural fibroids have similar amounts of *HOXA10* mRNA expression as control patients without fibroids [38]. Stromal expression of HOXA10 protein, via immunohistochemistry, is also differentially affected by submucosal versus intramural fibroids [40]. Endometrial biopsy specimens from directly over a submucosal fibroid and from nonadjacent endometria remote from the submucosal fibroid have lower levels of stromal HOXA10 protein expression compared to controls and patients with intramural fibroids [40]. There is no difference in HOXA10 stromal expression between controls and patients with intramural fibroids [40]. It appears that submucosal fibroids have a global effect on endometrial receptivity through stromal expression of HOXA10. These findings provide a possible mechanism by which submucosal fibroids exert a more profound effect on fertility compared to other fibroid subtypes.

Angiogenic and Vascular Factors

Angiogenesis and vascular development are critical for successful implantation. As fibroids grow, they induce vascular changes in the uterine architecture that may impede or hinder implantation. Molecular changes induced by fibroid growth can lead to an increase in the number of blood vessels and abnormal vascular function. Certain angiogenic factors such as basic fibroblast growth factor (bFGF) play a key role in fibroid growth and could potentially interfere with embryo implantation [41].

The bFGF is highly mitogenic and can induce angiogenesis *in vivo* [42]. This growth factor and its receptor are expressed in the human myometrium and endometrium [43]. Furthermore, bFGF has been shown to be stored in the extracellular matrix (ECM) and can initiate remodeling of the ECM, which is an important step in angiogenesis. Fibroids are characterized by having large amounts of ECM, within which are large amounts of bFGF [44]. Fibroids are therefore a large reservoir for bFGF, which can impact endometrial vasculature through a paracrine endocrine effect. A study by Anania et al. compared the expression of bFGF receptor (FGFR1) between women with fibroids and those without. The study found that in women with no fibroids, there was a suppression of stromal FGR1 expression during the early luteal phase, which was not observed in those women with fibroids [45]. The time coincides with embryo apposition and implantation. This finding is suggestive that the abnormal expression of bFGF and its receptors induced by fibroids may alter endometrial WOI.

Fibroids also possess an antiangiogenic profile when compared to normal myometrium. Fibroids have been shown to have higher amounts of antiangiogenic factors, such as collagen $4\alpha2$ (COL4A2), and lower expression of angiogenic promoters, such as connective tissue growth factor (CTGF) and cysteine-rich angiogenic inducer 61 (CYR-61) [46]. Together these create an antiangiogenic environment that may impact embryo receptivity and implantation in sites close to the fibroid.

Immunologic and Inflammatory Factors

Endometrial decidualization, promoted by increasing progesterone levels during the luteal phase, leads to the release of vascular endothelial growth factor (VEGF) and prostaglandins. The increase in vessel permeability induced by these two substances leads to the extravasation of polymorphonuclear cells from circulation. The cells, in turn, release various cytokines that have been shown to play a role in implantation, including leukemia inhibitory factor (LIF), interleukin-11 (IL-11), and transforming growth factor β (TGF-β). The presence of fibroids can alter the concentration of these cytokines, which may impact endometrial receptivity.

Both LIF and IL-11 act through the same gp130 signaling pathway [7,47]. Inactivation of this pathway has been associated with implantation failure in murine models [48]. Mice that are LIF deficient have recurrent implantation failure secondary to poor endometrial decidualization. Embryos from these defective mice are able to implant in wild-type mice [49]. Clinically, dysregulation of LIF expression during the secretory phase has been associated with unexplained infertility and recurrent pregnancy loss [50]. Peak LIF expression in humans coincides with the WOI. In the presence of submucosal fibroids, this increase in LIF expression is blunted [51]. Therefore, the presence of fibroids may prevent the release of cytokines, which are essential for implantation.

IL-11 promotes sustained endometrial decidualization. Murine studies have shown that mice that are IL-11 deficient experience pregnancy loss by the eighth day due to an inability to sustain decidualization [52]. In humans, IL-11 is also thought to aid trophoblast invasion [53]. The expression of IL-11 is diminished during the WOI in women with submucosal fibroids [51]. The diminished expression can affect the embryo's ability to implant.

The TGF-β isoforms are cytokines that play a key role in tissue morphogenesis and growth. Fibroids secrete high levels of the β3 isoforms during the secretory phase. These high levels induce a resistance of endometrial stromal cells to bone morphogenic protein 2 (BMP-2), which is known to play a role in effective decidualization and implantation [54]. In BMP-2 knockout mice, defective implantation leads to early pregnancy loss [55,56]. Levels of TGF-β seem to be correlated with fibroid size given that decreased levels are seen when fibroids shrink in response to gonadotropin-releasing hormone agonist therapy [57].

Natural killer (NK) cells and macrophages are among the immune cells released into the endometrium during the secretory phase in response to a rise in VEGF and prostaglandins [58]. NK cells are present during the WOI [59]. NK cells produce VEGF and placental growth factor, which regulate maternal-uterine vasculature remodeling and trophoblast invasion [60]. In knockout NK mice, pregnancies are complicated by miscarriages, severe growth restriction, and preeclampsia [61]. During the secretory phase, the endometria of women with fibroids tend to have an increase in macrophages and a decreased number of NK cells [62]. This may hinder endometrial receptivity to implantation.

Impact on Gene Expression

Fibroids can impact endometrial gene expression through varying means (Table 3.2). As introduced earlier in this section, fibroids can alter gene expression indirectly by increasing the secretion of the cytokine TGF-β3, which then causes the downregulation of BMPR-2 expression within the endometrium [54,57]. Direct regulation of gene expression by fibroids can also occur and appears to be spatially regulated. The homeobox genes are critical for embryo implantation and have been discussed in detail.

TABLE 3.2

Endometrial Genes Dysregulated by Fibroids

Gene Name	Regulation	Reference
HOXA10	Decreased expression with submucosal fibroids (mediated by BMP2); increased expression after myomectomy of intramural fibroid	[40,63]
HOXA11	Increased expression after myomectomy of intramural fibroid	[63]
LIF	Blunted expression with submucosal fibroids	[51]
IL11	Decreased expression with submucosal fibroids	[51]
BMPR2	Decreased expression as a result of increased TGF-β3, induced BMP2 resistance results in downregulation of BMPR2	[54,57]
BTEB1	Decreased expression with submucosal fibroids	[40]
ITGB3	Increased expression after myomectomy of intramural fibroid, although not significant	[63]

The presence of submucosal fibroids but not intramural fibroids decreases the expression of HOXA10. In contrast to Rackow and Taylor [40], Unlu et al. found the reverse to be true [63]. They investigated genes known to be important for endometrial receptivity (*HOXA10*, *HOXA11*, and *ITGAV*) in infertile women with either submucosal fibroids, intramural fibroids (noncavitary distorting), or a uterine septum before and after myomectomy compared to controls [63]. There was a trend in decreased mRNA expression in *HOXA10*, *HOXA11*, and *ITGAV* in women with submucosal or intramural fibroids that was not significant compared to controls. However, in women with intramural fibroids after myomectomy, there was a significant 12.8-fold and 9-fold increased expression of *HOXA10* and *HOXA11*, respectively. Although nonsignificant, there was also a 26-fold increase in *LIF* expression and 15.9-fold increase in *ITGB3* expression. Together their data suggest that there is a positive regulatory effect of gene expression after myomectomy of intramural fibroids. Conversely, they did not find a significant increase in mRNA expression after myomectomy in women with submucosal fibroids [63].

In another study evaluating intramural fibroids with noncavitary involvement, Horcajada et al. in 2008 performed gene expression analysis on endometrial tissue of women with intramural fibroids compared to controls without [36]. They identified that 3 of the 25 genes (*GPx3*, placental protein 14, and aldehyde dehydrogenase 3 family, member *B2* genes) related to the WOI were dysregulated in women with intramural fibroids greater than 5 cm, suggesting that larger fibroids may have an effect on endometrial gene expression. However, because the number of genes dysregulated was limited to three, they concluded that fibroids without endometrial cavity involvement did not affect genes involved in implantation. Although studies have shown that fibroids do alter gene expression within the endometrium, there are conflicting data regarding whether submucosal or noncavitary intramural fibroids have a greater impact. Additional studies are needed in order to further elucidate these findings.

Conclusion

In summary, there are multiple mechanisms by which fibroids can alter endometrial receptivity. Key mechanisms include mechanical disruption by directly blocking gamete and embryo transport as well as increased uterine peristaltic activity due to higher levels of estrogen from increased expression of aromatase enzyme found in fibroid cells. Additionally, fibroids can cause an upregulation or downregulation of specific genes, such as *HOX10A*, leading to changes in cytokines and growth factors like bFGF, LIF, IL-11, and TGF-β, which may also impact endometrial receptivity.

Research and Future Therapeutics

In the age of personalized medicine and targeted genomics, analysis of the endometrium for optimal receptivity in the presence of fibroids is an area of future research. The ERA test, a microarray analysis of 238 genes from tissue obtained by endometrial biopsy, has been developed to assist in identifying the WOI in patients undergoing IVF to optimize the timing of embryo transfer [23,64]. Though promising, the ERA is a relatively new diagnostic tool that is currently undergoing multicenter clinical trials, and additional research outcomes are required to validate its use. Perhaps in the future this technology can also be applied to assess the endometrial receptivity of uteri affected by fibroids.

REFERENCES

1. Baird DD, Dunson DB, Hill MC et al. High cumulative incidence of uterine leiomyoma in black and white women: Ultrasound evidence. *Am J Obstet Gynecol.* 2003;188(1):100–7.
2. Pritts EA, Parker WH, and Olive DL. Fibroids and infertility: An updated systematic review of the evidence. *Fertil Steril.* 2009;91(4):1215–23.
3. Bulun SE. Uterine fibroids. *N Engl J Med.* 2013;369(14):1344–55.
4. Bulletti C, Ziegler D, Levi Setti P et al. Myomas, pregnancy outcome, and *in vitro* fertilization. *Ann N Y Acad Sci.* 2004;1034:84–92.

5. Donnez J and Jadoul P. What are the implications of myomas on fertility? A need for a debate? *Hum Reprod.* 2002;17(6):1424–30.

6. Whynott RM, Vaught KCC, and Segars JH. The effect of uterine fibroids on infertility: A systematic review. *Semin Reprod Med.* 2017;35(6):523–32.

7. Dey SK, Lim H, Das SK et al. Molecular cues to implantation. *Endocr Rev.* 2004;25(3):341–73.

8. Singh M, Chaudhry P, and Asselin E. Bridging endometrial receptivity and implantation: Network of hormones, cytokines, and growth factors. *J Endocrinol.* 2011;210(1):5–14.

9. Dimitriadis E, White CA, Jones RL et al. Cytokines, chemokines and growth factors in endometrium related to implantation. *Hum Reprod Update.* 2005;11(6):613–30.

10. Gellersen B and Brosens JJ. Cyclic decidualization of the human endometrium in reproductive health and failure. *Endocr Rev.* 2014;35(6):851–905.

11. Noyes RW, Hertig AT, and Rock J. Dating the endometrial biopsy. *Am J Obstet Gynecol.* 1975;122(2):262–3.

12. Myers ER, Silva S, Barnhart K et al. Interobserver and intraobserver variability in the histological dating of the endometrium in fertile and infertile women. *Fertil Steril.* 2004;82(5):1278–82.

13. Demiral İ, Doğan M, Baştu E et al. Genomic, proteomic and lipidomic evaluation of endometrial receptivity. *Turk J Obstet Gynecol.* 2015;12(4):237–43.

14. Kao LC, Tulac S, Lobo S et al. Global gene profiling in human endometrium during the window of implantation. *Endocrinology.* 2002;143(6):2119–38.

15. Carson DD, Lagow E, Thathiah A et al. Changes in gene expression during the early to mid-luteal (receptive phase) transition in human endometrium detected by high-density microarray screening. *Mol Hum Reprod.* 2002;8(9):871–9.

16. Borthwick JM, Charnock-Jones DS, Tom BD et al. Determination of the transcript profile of human endometrium. *Mol Hum Reprod.* 2003;9(1):19–33.

17. Riesewijk A, Martín J, van Os R et al. Gene expression profiling of human endometrial receptivity on days LH+2 versus LH+7 by microarray technology. *Mol Hum Reprod.* 2003;9(5):253–64.

18. Mirkin S, Arslan M, Churikov D et al. In search of candidate genes critically expressed in the human endometrium during the window of implantation. *Hum Reprod.* 2005;20(8):2104–17.

19. Ponnampalam AP, Weston GC, Trajstman AC et al. Molecular classification of human endometrial cycle stages by transcriptional profiling. *Mol Hum Reprod.* 2004;10(12):879–93.

20. Talbi S, Hamilton AE, Vo KC et al. Molecular phenotyping of human endometrium distinguishes menstrual cycle phases and underlying biological processes in normo-ovulatory women. *Endocrinology.* 2006;147(3):1097–121.

21. Horcajadas JA, Pellicer A, and Simón C. Wide genomic analysis of human endometrial receptivity: New times, new opportunities. *Hum Reprod Update.* 2007;13(1):77–86.

22. Díaz-Gimeno P, Horcajadas JA, Martínez-Conejero JA et al. A genomic diagnostic tool for human endometrial receptivity based on the transcriptomic signature. *Fertil Steril.* 2011;95(1):60.e15.

23. Ruiz-Alonso M, Blesa D, Díaz-Gimeno P et al. The endometrial receptivity array for diagnosis and personalized embryo transfer as a treatment for patients with repeated implantation failure. *Fertil Steril.* 2013;100(3):818–24.

24. Horcajadas JA, Mínguez P, Dopazo J et al. Controlled ovarian stimulation induces a functional genomic delay of the endometrium with potential clinical implications. *J Clin Endocrinol Metab.* 2008;93(11):4500–10.

25. Chalmers JA. Fibromyoma of the fallopian tube. *J Obstet Gynaecol Br Emp.* 1948;55(2):155–8.

26. Maltaris T, Dittrich R, Widjaja W et al. The role of oestradiol in the uterine peristalsis in the perfused swine uterus. *Reprod Domest Anim.* 2006;41(6):522–6.

27. Kissler S, Siebzehnruebl E, Kohl J et al. Uterine contractility and directed sperm transport assessed by hysterosalpingoscintigraphy (HSSG) and intrauterine pressure (IUP) measurement. *Acta Obstet Gynecol Scand.* 2004;83(4):369–74.

28. Fujiwara T, Togashi K, Yamaoka T et al. Kinematics of the uterus: Cine mode MR imaging. *Radiographics.* 2004;24(1):e19.

29. Fanchin R, Ayoubi JM, Righini C et al. Uterine contractility decreases at the time of blastocyst transfers. *Hum Reprod.* 2001;16(6):1115–9.

30. Fanchin R, Righini C, Olivennes F et al. Uterine contractions at the time of embryo transfer alter pregnancy rates after in-vitro fertilization. *Hum Reprod.* 1998;13(7):1968–74.

31. Yoshino O, Hayashi T, Osuga Y et al. Decreased pregnancy rate is linked to abnormal uterine peristalsis caused by intramural fibroids. *Hum Reprod*. 2010;25(10):2475–9.
32. Yoshino O, Nishii O, Osuga Y et al. Myomectomy decreases abnormal uterine peristalsis and increases pregnancy rate. *J Minim Invasive Gynecol*. 2012;19(1):63–7.
33. Folkerd EJ, Newton CJ, Davidson K et al. Aromatase activity in uterine leiomyomata. *J Steroid Biochem*. 1984;20(5):1195–200.
34. Bulun SE, Simpson ER, and Word RA. Expression of the CYP19 gene and its product aromatase cytochrome P450 in human uterine leiomyoma tissues and cells in culture. *J Clin Endocrinol Metab*. 1994;78(3):736–43.
35. Patterson-Keels LM, Selvaggi SM, Haefner HK et al. Morphologic assessment of endometrium overlying submucosal leiomyomas. *J Reprod Med*. 1994;39(8):579–84.
36. Horcajadas JA, Goyri E, Higón MA et al. Endometrial receptivity and implantation are not affected by the presence of uterine intramural leiomyomas: A clinical and functional genomics analysis. *J Clin Endocrinol Metab*. 2008;93(9):3490–8.
37. Brosens J, Campo R, Gordts S et al. Submucous and outer myometrium leiomyomas are two distinct clinical entities. *Fertil Steril*. 2003;79(6):1452–4.
38. Horne AW and Critchley HO. The effect of uterine fibroids on embryo implantation. *Semin Reprod Med*. 2007;25(6):483–9.
39. Satokata I, Benson G, and Maas R. Sexually dimorphic sterility phenotypes in Hoxa10-deficient mice. *Nature*. 1995;374(6521):460–3.
40. Rackow BW and Taylor HS. Submucosal uterine leiomyomas have a global effect on molecular determinants of endometrial receptivity. *Fertil Steril*. 2010;93(6):2027–34.
41. Di Lieto A, De Falco M, Pollio F et al. Clinical response, vascular change, and angiogenesis in gonadotropin-releasing hormone analogue-treated women with uterine myomas. *J Soc Gynecol Investig*. 2005;12(2):123–8.
42. Folkman J and Klagsbrun M. Angiogenic factors. *Science*. 1987;235(4787):442–7.
43. Salat-Baroux J, Romain S, Alvarez S et al. Biochemical and immunohistochemical multiparametric analysis of steroid receptors and growth factor receptors in human normal endometrium in spontaneous cycles and after the induction of ovulation. *Hum Reprod*. 1994;9(2):200–8.
44. Mangrulkar RS, Ono M, Ishikawa M et al. Isolation and characterization of heparin-binding growth factors in human leiomyomas and normal myometrium. *Biol Reprod*. 1995;53(3):636–46.
45. Anania CA, Stewart EA, Quade BJ et al. Expression of the fibroblast growth factor receptor in women with leiomyomas and abnormal uterine bleeding. *Mol Hum Reprod*. 1997;3(8):685–91.
46. Weston G, Trajstman AC, Gargett CE et al. Fibroids display an anti-angiogenic gene expression profile when compared with adjacent myometrium. *Mol Hum Reprod*. 2003;9(9):541–9.
47. Kishimoto T, Tanaka T, Yoshida K et al. Cytokine signal transduction through a homo- or heterodimer of gp130. *Ann N Y Acad Sci*. 1995;766:224–34.
48. Ernst M, Inglese M, Waring P et al. Defective gp130-mediated signal transducer and activator of transcription (STAT) signaling results in degenerative joint disease, gastrointestinal ulceration, and failure of uterine implantation. *J Exp Med*. 2001;194(2):189–203.
49. Stewart CL, Kaspar P, Brunet LJ et al. Blastocyst implantation depends on maternal expression of leukaemia inhibitory factor. *Nature*. 1992;359(6390):76–9.
50. Hambartsoumian E. Endometrial leukemia inhibitory factor (LIF) as a possible cause of unexplained infertility and multiple failures of implantation. *Am J Reprod Immunol*. 1998;39(2):137–43.
51. Hasegawa E, Ito H, Hasegawa F et al. Expression of leukemia inhibitory factor in the endometrium in abnormal uterine cavities during the implantation window. *Fertil Steril*. 2012;97(4):953–8.
52. Robb L, Li R, Hartley L et al. Infertility in female mice lacking the receptor for interleukin 11 is due to a defective uterine response to implantation. *Nat Med*. 1998;4(3):303–8.
53. Zenclussen AC and Hämmerling GJ. Cellular regulation of the uterine microenvironment that enables embryo implantation. *Front Immunol*. 2015;6:321.
54. Doherty LF and Taylor HS. Leiomyoma-derived transforming growth factor-beta impairs bone morphogenetic protein-2-mediated endometrial receptivity. *Fertil Steril*. 2015;103(3):845–52.
55. Li Q, Kannan A, Das A et al. WNT4 acts downstream of BMP2 and functions via β-catenin signaling pathway to regulate human endometrial stromal cell differentiation. *Endocrinology*. 2013;154(1):446–57.

56. Lee KY, Jeong J, Wang J et al. Bmp2 is critical for the murine uterine decidual response. *Mol Cell Biol.* 2007;27(15):5468–78.
57. Dou Q, Zhao Y, Tarnuzzer RW et al. Suppression of transforming growth factor-beta (TGF beta) and TGF beta receptor messenger ribonucleic acid and protein expression in leiomyomata in women receiving gonadotropin-releasing hormone agonist therapy. *J Clin Endocrinol Metab.* 1996;81(9):3222–30.
58. Miura S, Khan KN, Kitajima M et al. Differential infiltration of macrophages and prostaglandin production by different uterine leiomyomas. *Hum Reprod.* 2006;21(10):2545–54.
59. Lee SK, Kim CJ, Kim D et al. Immune cells in the female reproductive tract. *Immune Netw.* 2015;15(1):16–26.
60. Tayade C, Hilchie D, He H et al. Genetic deletion of placenta growth factor in mice alters uterine NK cells. *J Immunol.* 2007;178(7):4267–75.
61. King A. Uterine leukocytes and decidualization. *Hum Reprod Update.* 2000;6(1):28–36.
62. Kitaya K and Yasuo T. Leukocyte density and composition in human cycling endometrium with uterine fibroids. *Hum Immunol.* 2010;71(2):158–63.
63. Unlu C, Celik O, Celik N et al. Expression of endometrial receptivity genes increase after myomectomy of intramural leiomyomas not distorting the endometrial cavity. *Reprod Sci.* 2016;23(1):31–41.
64. Miravet-Valenciano JA, Rincon-Bertolin A, Vilella F et al. Understanding and improving endometrial receptivity. *Curr Opin Obstet Gynecol.* 2015;27(3):187–92.
65. Taylor HS, Pal L, Seli E, eds, Conception – Sperm and egg transport, fertilization, implantation and early embryogenesis. In: *Speroff's Clinicl Gynecologic Endocrinology and Infertility*, 9th edn, Wolters Kluwer, Philadelphia, 2020: 174–95.

4

Uterine Fibroids and Recurrent Pregnancy Loss

Natasha K. Simula and Mohamed A. Bedaiwy

CONTENTS

Introduction

Uterine fibroids are the most common benign tumor of the female reproductive tract. Prevalence in the general reproductive-age population has been estimated at 5.4%, with increasing prevalence in older age groups [1]. The prevalence in pregnant women has been reported at 0.65%–10.6% [2–6]. Fibroids are known to be associated with adverse pregnancy outcomes, such as malpresentation [3], placental abruption [5,6], preterm delivery [2,3,5,7], cesarean section [2,3,5], as well as increased blood loss with delivery and need for postpartum blood transfusion [7]. Fibroids may also be associated with infertility, spontaneous abortion (SA), and recurrent pregnancy loss (RPL), although this association is not as well established.

The type of fibroid is important in this setting. Subserosal fibroids are currently not thought to contribute to pregnancy loss or infertility, and myomectomy for subserosal fibroids is not generally offered as a treatment for women trying to achieve a pregnancy. Submucosal fibroids are associated with lower fertility rates, but their role in recurrent pregnancy loss is still under investigation [8], as we discuss in this chapter. Intramural fibroids that distort the cavity are also thought to affect fertility, but even those intramural fibroids that do not distort the cavity may negatively affect early pregnancy outcomes [3,8–11]. Unfortunately, a lot of the studies do not indicate the type of fibroid participants have, so drawing general conclusions from these studies can be difficult. Number and location of fibroids are also not discussed in many studies, and these are all characteristics that studies moving forward should report. There is some evidence that at least the number of fibroids may matter, with higher SA rates in women with multiple fibroids compared to women with a single fibroid [12].

Fibroids and Pregnancy Loss

The pathophysiology of fibroids and pregnancy loss as well as recurrent pregnancy loss is not well understood. Buttram et al. [13] published the first study linking fibroids to pregnancy loss in 1981. They performed a literature review of published myomectomy cases and included 59 cases of their own, and they showed that SA rates decreased from 41% to 19% after myomectomy. They suggested that miscarriage may occur in women with fibroids because of uterine irritability and contractility, and/or changes in the endometrial stroma and vasculature that may reduce placental blood flow leading to miscarriage [13]. Fibroids may also degenerate in pregnancy causing an inflammatory reaction with prostaglandin release and resulting contractions and miscarriage [2].

Several observational studies since Buttram et al's. paper in 1981 have shown similar results that women with fibroids may have higher rates of pregnancy loss than women without fibroids. The largest study published to date was a prospective, age-matched, cohort study that included 143 women with fibroids diagnosed on first-trimester ultrasound compared with 715 women without fibroids. The risk for SA in women with fibroids was significantly higher than in women without fibroids (14% versus 7.6%) [12]. However, two older studies failed to find a statistically significant difference in SA rates when studying a general pregnant population of 12,708 women (492 with uterine myomas) [6] as well as in a population of 290 patients undergoing *in vitro* fertilization (IVF) [14].

Klatsky et al. [3] performed a systematic review of 20 studies, which included the three studies mentioned earlier, and found a statistically significant increase in the cumulative SA rate in women with submucosal fibroids ($n = 15$; 46.7% SA rate) compared with controls ($n = 151$; 21.9%; odds ratio [OR] 3.85; confidence interval [CI] 1.12–13.27). The correlation was weaker, although still significant, for women with intramural fibroids and a documented first-trimester ultrasound. The cumulative SA rate for women with an intramural fibroid was 20.4% ($n = 719$) versus 12.9% in women without fibroids ($n = 2258$; OR 1.82; CI 1.43–2.30) [3].

A recent systematic review of 18 studies that reported pregnancy loss outcomes also found a statistically significant increase in SA rate in women with fibroids compared with women without fibroids (relative risk [RR] 1.68; CI 1.37–2.05). Subgroup analyses comparing controls to women with submucosal fibroids and women with intramural fibroids also showed statistically significant higher rates of SA in both groups (RR 1.68 for women with submucous fibroids; RR 1.89 for women with intramural fibroids) [8].

However, an even more recent systematic review and meta-analysis published in 2017 included a population of 21,829 pregnancies (1394 women with fibroids) and adjusted for possible confounders (e.g., age, race, alcohol use, parity, history of prior terminations). It was found that there was no statistically significant increase in SA rates in women with fibroids compared to women without fibroids (RR 0.82; CI 0.68–0.98). Studies that included women with RPL, infertility, or assisted reproduction technology (ART) use were excluded from this meta-analysis [15]. Overall, the data available are conflicting, and a possible relationship between uterine fibroids and pregnancy loss in the general pregnant population is yet to be determined.

Fibroids and Recurrent Pregnancy Loss

There are very few studies of the prevalence of fibroids in the RPL population. One prospective cohort study that included 23 patients with otherwise unexplained primary RPL found one patient (4.3%) with a submucosal fibroid on hysteroscopy [16]. The prevalence in another study in which 150 patients had hysteroscopy found two patients (1.3%) with submucosal fibroids, both of which had three or more recurrent SAs [17]. Saravelos et al. studied a group of 966 women with three or more recurrent SAs and found an 8.2% ($n = 70$) prevalence of fibroids, including both submucosal and intramural/subserosal fibroids [10].

A meta-analysis performed by Russo et al. in 2016 included three studies with a total of 711 participants undergoing RPL investigations. The prevalence of submucosal fibroids and fibroids distorting the cavity was 4.08%. Prevalence was higher in women with a higher number of losses [18]. However, the authors indicate that the relationship between fibroids and RPL is yet to be established, as none of the studies that have been done had an appropriate control group.

More recently, a study performed in an RPL clinic in Australia assessed uterine anatomy by three-dimensional (3D) ultrasonography in 190 women and found a fibroid prevalence of 15%, although the types of fibroids were not noted. Fibroids were more common in women older than 35 years old [19]. Lastly, anatomic workup by office hysteroscopy in 200 women attending an RPL clinic in Egypt revealed a prevalence of 7.5% for submucosal fibroids [20], but again, findings like these are difficult to interpret without an appropriate control group. Based on these data, it appears that the overall prevalence of fibroids in the RPL population is somewhere between 4% and 15%.

Evaluation of Anatomic Factors in Recurrent Pregnancy Loss

The approach to RPL varies between centers, but a comprehensive workup usually involves assessment of uterine anatomy, as well as endocrine, autoimmune, and cytogenetic factors, as per the American Society of Reproductive Medicine (ASRM) 2012 guideline on recurrent pregnancy loss [21]. Evaluation for antiphospholipid antibody syndrome and thrombophilias is restricted to patients who meet certain special criteria. Despite extensive investigations, approximately 50%–75% of patients will have unexplained RPL [21].

Uterine anatomic factors are implicated in approximately 12.6% of cases of RPL [21] and include both congenital and acquired causes. Examples of congenital müllerian anomalies that may contribute to RPL include uterine septum, bicornuate, unicornuate, and arcuate uteri. Examples of acquired factors include fibroids, polyps, and Asherman syndrome from uterine synechiae. The ASRM recommends assessment of the uterine cavity by hysterosalpingography, magnetic resonance imaging (MRI), or 3D ultrasound [21]. However, hysteroscopy is also widely used and is considered the gold standard for diagnosis of uterine anomalies [17,20,22,23]. Table 4.1 lists the diagnostic imaging modalities and their reported sensitivity and specificity.

Hysteroscopy allows direct visualization of the uterine cavity and any submucosal lesion that may be present. It can be performed easily in the office as a diagnostic tool, and under conscious sedation or in the operating room for concurrent diagnosis and treatment. However, as with hysterosalpingography (HSG) discussed later, it does not assess the external contour of the uterus, so it may miss non-cavity-distorting intramural fibroids as well as other congenital uterine anomalies. One study comparing hysteroscopy with pathology diagnosis of hysterectomy specimens found a sensitivity of 82% and specificity of 87% for hysteroscopic diagnosis of submucous fibroids [24]. Figure 4.1 shows an example of an International Federation of Gynecology and Obstetrics (FIGO) type 2 fibroid of the anterior wall.

Two-dimensional (2D) transvaginal ultrasonography (TVUS) is an accurate method of diagnosing the presence of fibroids with a sensitivity of 99% and specificity of 86%. However, 2D TVUS is not as good as MRI, for example, in mapping and characterizing type and location of fibroids, especially in women

TABLE 4.1

Sensitivity and Specificity of Diagnostic Modalities for Evaluation of Uterine Fibroids

Diagnostic Modality	Sensitivity (%)	Specificity (%)
Hysteroscopy	82[a]	87[a]
2D Ultrasound	99	86
3D Ultrasound	68.2[a]	91.5[a]
Hysterosalpingography (HSG)	50[a]	82.5[a]
Saline infusion sonohystogram (SIS)	90[a]	89[a]
Magnetic resonance imaging (MRI)	100	91

[a] Sensitivity and specificity reported for identification of submucous fibroids.

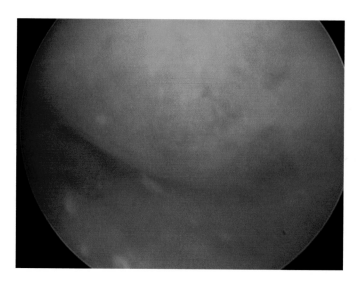

FIGURE 4.1 Example of a FIGO type 2 fibroid diagnosed by hysteroscopy in a patient with recurrent pregnancy loss.

with more than four fibroids [25]. Two-dimensional TVUS also does not perform as well as an MRI in detection of submucosal fibroids (TVUS: sensitivity 83% and specificity 90%; MRI: sensitivity 100% and specificity 91%) [24]. The main advantage of 2D TVUS is how readily available it is for clinicians, but it does have its limitations with low sensitivity in the detection of other uterine anomalies, such as congenital uterine anomalies (sensitivity 56%; specificity 99%) [26], and the depth of penetration of a 2D TVUS may not reach a very large or fundal fibroid, and transabdominal ultrasound may be necessary as a complementary technique [27]. The advantage of 3D ultrasound over 2D ultrasound is that it displays an image of the uterus in the longitudinal, transverse, and coronal planes, giving a better assessment of the external uterine contour in addition to the uterine body and endometrial cavity [19,26–28]. A prospective observational cross-sectional study comparing 3D ultrasound with hysteroscopic findings in 61 patients found a sensitivity of 68.2% and specificity of 91.5% for 3D ultrasound in the detection of intrauterine pathology. All submucous fibroids were detected by 3D ultrasound, but it was not as good at detection of endometrial polyps, missing 7 out of 18 polyps seen on hysteroscopy [28].

HSG is a procedure in which a radiopaque solution is instilled into the uterus while fluoroscopy is being performed. It can be added to 2D TVUS in the assessment of the uterine cavity; however, it is most useful in assessing tubal patency in an infertility workup. Sensitivity and specificity are low in diagnosing intrauterine pathology, and HSG should not be used as the main diagnostic modality for uterine pathology [29]. Elsokkary et al. performed HSG and hysteroscopy in 200 women with a history of RPL and found that 13.3% of women (2 out of 15) had a normal HSG when in fact there was a submucous fibroid identified on hysteroscopy [20].

Sonohysterography or saline infusion sonohystogram (SIS) involves the injection of saline into the uterine cavity while performing a 2D TVUS. In many centers, this is a more convenient option over HSG as it can be performed in the office by an experienced gynecologist rather than having to schedule the procedure at a radiology clinic [27]. SIS has a sensitivity of 90% and specificity of 89% for submucosal fibroid detection [24], but it is not an appropriate modality in assessing non-cavity-distorting intramural fibroids.

MRI is expensive and not always readily available, but the sensitivity (100%) and specificity (91%) in detecting fibroids are superior to other techniques, including for submucous fibroids [24]. It is also useful in delineating the location and number of fibroids [24,25], which is especially important when planning a complex surgical procedure such as a laparoscopic, robotic, or open myomectomy [9,27,30]. MRI is also ideal to distinguish adenomyosis from fibroids in equivocal cases [27]. Figure 4.2 shows an example of a single posterior intramural fibroid and of a multifibroid uterus where fibroid mapping by MRI preoperatively would be especially helpful.

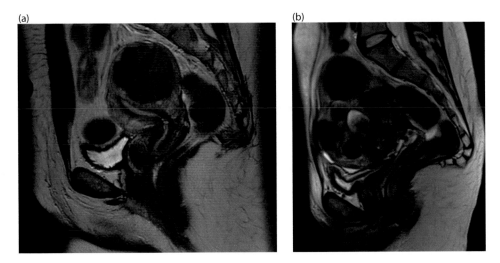

FIGURE 4.2   Sagittal magnetic resonance imaging of a single non-cavity-distorting posterior fibroid (a) and a multifibroid uterus with cavity-distorting fibroids (b) in two different patients with recurrent pregnancy loss.

Treatment

Once a fibroid has been diagnosed in a woman with RPL, the question becomes whether she should be treated or not. The literature on both medical and noninvasive radiological and surgical management strategies is reviewed here. However, medical management is not considered definitive treatment for fibroids and is not recommended when patients are trying to conceive. It is generally accepted that submucous and cavity-distorting intramural fibroids should be removed, and subserosal fibroids should be left alone [9–11,31,32]. Expectant management is also an option but is usually only considered in women with large intramural fibroids that do not distort the cavity [9] or for women with subserosal fibroids [32]. Table 4.2 lists the treatment options and for whom each option should be recommended.

Medical Management

Hormonal medical therapies that are available for treatment of fibroids are contraindicated for use in pregnancy and in women who are trying to conceive. Medications are usually taken for symptomatic

TABLE 4.2

Treatment Options for Women with Fibroids and Recurrent Pregnancy Loss

Treatment	Indications
Expectant management	Patient choice FIGO type 4, 5, 6, and 7
Medical management: ulipristal acetate (UPA)	Not indicated for women planning a pregnancy but some evidence that it is safe to conceive after use
Uterine artery embolization (UAE)	Not indicated for women planning a pregnancy
Magnetic resonance–guided focused ultrasound surgery (MRgFUS)	Not indicated for women planning a pregnancy but some evidence that it is safe to conceive after procedure
Ultrasound-guided radiofrequency ablation (RFA)	Not indicated for women planning a pregnancy but some evidence that it is safe to conceive after procedure
Hysteroscopic myomectomy	FIGO type 0 and I
Abdominal or laparoscopic myomectomy	FIGO type 2 and 2-5 FIGO type 4, 5, and 6 measuring greater than 5 cm

management of abnormal uterine bleeding and bulk symptoms. These include gonadotropin-releasing hormone (GnRH) agonists such as leuprolide, GnRH analogues such as goserelin, selective estrogen receptor modulators (SERMs) such as raloxifene, and selective progesterone receptor modulators (SPRMs) such as ulipristal acetate (UPA). These therapies are aimed at suppression of estrogen and progesterone effects on fibroids, but they also affect ovulation and the endometrium, and in turn can affect implantation and placentation [9].

Although UPA is contraindicated in pregnancy (and is also used as emergency contraception although at a higher dose than that used for fibroids), there is some evidence that pregnancy following UPA use may be safe. A systematic review of pregnancies after UPA use combined 24 pregnancies published in the literature with their own case series of 47 pregnancies, for a total of 71 pregnancies examined [33]. Five patients inadvertently became pregnant while taking UPA, resulting in three live births, one SA, and one therapeutic abortion. The remaining patients became pregnant approximately 2–4.5 months after UPA use. Forty-seven pregnancies occurred without an interval myomectomy, and for the whole group of 71 pregnancies, there were 50 live births. The SA rate was 27% with a total of 19 SAs [33].

Procedural Options

Uterine artery embolization is used to impair major blood flow to growing fibroids and is an outpatient procedure performed by an interventional radiologist. The risks of this procedure include the need for retreatment, dyspareunia due to inadvertent embolization of the vaginal artery, decreased ovarian reserve, infertility, and miscarriage [34]. Due to these risks, this procedure is generally considered contraindicated in women who wish to conceive [9,32,34].

Magnetic resonance–guided focused ultrasound surgery (MRgFUS) is a relatively new, noninvasive method used to treat mostly intramural fibroids, but it has also been described for treatment of FIGO class I fibroids [35]. MRI is used to define the anatomy, and an ultrasound transducer is used to deliver pulses of energy that generate heat and induce coagulative necrosis of the fibroid. The procedure is lengthy, taking 3–5 hours to complete, and care must be taken not to injure adjacent structures that may be in the path of the transducer beam. Complications reported in the literature include skin burns, nerve damage, and visceral injury. As with uterine artery embolization, there is also a risk for needing retreatment [34].

Several case reports have been published of pregnancies after MRgFUS treatment, and they show positive pregnancy outcomes [36]. However, publication bias favoring publication of positive reports only limits the interpretation of the data, and the only conclusion that can be made is that pregnancy seems to be safe after treatment with MRgFUS. A randomized controlled trial (NCT00730886, clinicaltrials.gov) started in 2008 was terminated early due to lack of enrollment. Further studies are needed to evaluate the impact of MRgFUS on pregnancy outcomes and specifically in pregnancy loss before it becomes a standard treatment offered to women wishing to conceive.

Ultrasound-guided radiofrequency ablation (RFA) is a new technique that involves delivery of alternating current through an RFA device. This is done under direct laparoscopic as well as ultrasound guidance using a laparoscopic ultrasound transducer. The RFA device is inserted into the fibroid, and the tissue is heated to up to 100°C, leading to coagulative necrosis [34]. This procedure has also been described using a transcervical approach with intrauterine sonography [37]. A retrospective observational study was published in 2017 which showed a pregnancy rate of 19.2% after treatment. Seventy eight out of 406 patients had a total of 80 pregnancies, with 71 live births and only 9 miscarriages. This suggests that perhaps pregnancy is safe after this treatment modality [38]. However, data are still very limited, and pregnancy is not recommended after ultrasound-guided RFA.

Hysteroscopic Myomectomy

Hysteroscopic myomectomy is performed for submucosal fibroids that are either entirely within the endometrial cavity or less than 50% intramural (FIGO classification type 0 and 1) [32]. Several studies have found that hysteroscopic myomectomy significantly decreases the rate of miscarriage, although these studies are observational and do not usually include control groups.

(a)   (b)

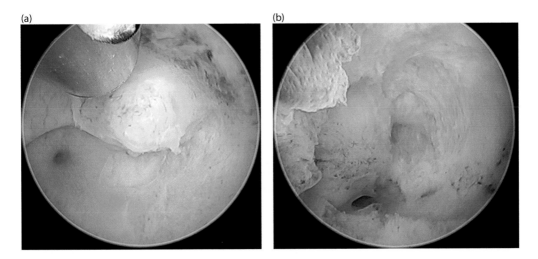

FIGURE 4.3   Left-sided FIGO type 1 fibroid in a patient with RPL before (a) and after (b) hysteroscopic resection.

Shokeir et al. demonstrated a significant decrease in first-trimester SAs from 61.6% to 26.3% in a cohort of 15 women with previous miscarriage who were followed prospectively for a mean time of 40 months [39]. A retrospective study of 101 women with recurrent miscarriage who underwent hysteroscopic myomectomy found similar results with a significant decrease in the first-trimester SA rate from 69.1% to 23.3% and second-trimester SA rate from 11.7% to 1.29% [40].

Saravelos et al. compared pregnancy outcomes between a group of 285 women with unexplained RPL and a group of 25 women with fibroids distorting the cavity who received myomectomy, as well as another group of 54 women with non-cavity-distorting fibroids who did not receive myomectomy. Myomectomies were mostly performed hysteroscopically except for in three patients who underwent open and laparoscopic myomectomy. There was a statistically significant decrease in midtrimester losses after myomectomy (21.7% before versus 0% after surgery) but no statistically significant difference in first-trimester losses. These women were not compared with the control group of women without fibroids. Women with intramural fibroids who were managed expectantly had a similar live birth rate (70.4%) as women with unexplained RPL (71.9%) after referral to clinic, which was improved from 20% live birth rate prior to clinic referral. Therefore, the authors conclude that women with intramural fibroids should be managed expectantly, and women with a history of midtrimester loss and cavity-distorting fibroids should be offered myomectomy. They also suggest that women with a history of first-trimester losses and cavity-distorting fibroids should be managed expectantly, as there was no statistically significant improvement in pregnancy outcomes in this group [10]. However, these general conclusions should be interpreted with caution as the data they is based on are merely observational.

Hysteroscopic myomectomy is a safe procedure that can be done in a surgical outpatient setting or with minimal anesthesia in an office setting depending on number and size of fibroids and should be offered to women with RPL who are found to have FIGO type 0, 1, and 2 fibroids. Figure 4.3 demonstrates an anterior FIGO type 1 fibroid before and after hysteroscopic resection.

Laparoscopic and Abdominal Myomectomy

The majority of published observational studies indicate that there may be a reduction in miscarriage rate after laparoscopic or open myomectomy for intramural fibroids. However, there have been no studies that focus solely on an RPL population.

One of the most cited reviews on this subject by Buttram et al. found a decrease in miscarriage rate from 41% to 19% with open myomectomy in a pooled review of 1941 cases [13]. The miscarriage rate also significantly declined from 57.1% to 13.8% in a study published in 2003 which included 25 patients who achieved a pregnancy after open or laparoscopic myomectomy [41]. Bernardi et al. followed 59 women after laparoscopic myomectomy for fibroids that were FIGO type 2-7 with a median of two fibroids removed per patient. The surgery was done for a variety of indications, including infertility, heavy bleeding, and dysmenorrhea, and patients were followed for approximately 6 years postoperatively. The miscarriage rate was also found to be lower after myomectomy (23%) compared to before myomectomy(43%) [42]. Similar results were also reported by Marchionni et al. [43] and Vercellini et al. [44] in studies including infertile women.

However, Casini et al. did not demonstrate a significant difference in miscarriage rates after myomectomy for intramural and subserosal fibroids in a study that included 181 participants with infertility. This study is unique in that they had an appropriate control group. Of the 181 participants, 92 patients had open or hysteroscopic myomectomy, and 89 patients were managed expectantly. Miscarriage rates were lower, although not statistically significant, in women who had hysteroscopic myomectomy for submucous fibroids (38.5%) compared with women who did not. However, miscarriage rates were no different in women who underwent myomectomy for intramural fibroids compared to those who did not have surgery [45]. These results are interesting and definitely add to the body of literature on the subject, but one must be careful in extrapolating findings from an infertile patient population to an RPL population.

In our RPL clinic, we recommend myomectomy for cavity-distorting intramural fibroids as well as fibroids that are larger than 5 cm, even if they are not cavity distorting, particularly in patients with recurrent euploid pregnancy loss with otherwise unexplained RPL. The decision between laparoscopy and laparotomy for myomectomy of intramural fibroids is based on number and diameter of fibroids. A laparoscopic approach is recommended if there is a single fibroid measuring less than 15 cm, two fibroids measuring less than 7.5 cm each, or if there are three fibroids measuring less than 5 cm each. If fibroids do not meet these criteria, lower transverse laparotomy is recommended [9].

Laparoscopic or open myomectomy is not without risks. Standard risks of surgery include significant blood loss, bowel injury, bladder injury [46], and wound infection [47]. In addition to standard surgical risks, such as anesthetic risk, postoperative venous thromboembolism, infection, bleeding, and injury to bowel, bladder, or ureter, there is also a small risk for uterine rupture in a subsequent labor [47], 21%–25% risk for fibroid recurrence [43,44], and risk for adhesions [44,48], which may lead to pain, bowel obstruction, and infertility [47]. Postoperative adhesions occur in higher frequency with posterior uterine incisions (94%) than with anterior uterine incisions (55%) [48]. Adhesion barriers are used by some surgeons, but the data on the benefit of these are inconclusive [39] and may actually indicate a lack of benefit in addition to added harm with increased rates of postoperative fever and ileus [49].

Conclusion

The body of evidence on the role of fibroids in recurrent pregnancy loss is growing, but there is a paucity of well-designed controlled trials to guide evidence-based management. Most studies are observational and lack proper control groups, making it difficult to draw strong conclusions. Future research in this area needs to include women without fibroids and women with untreated fibroids as controls, and other confounding factors need to be adjusted for as well, such as age, ethnicity, and primary versus secondary RPL. Studies also need to standardize the way fibroids are classified according to the FIGO classification system published in 2011 [50], and they should report the number and size of fibroids, so that results between studies can be better compared.

Evaluation for fibroids (and other congenital and acquired anomalies) should be made based on a combination of diagnostic modalities tailored to each patient. It should at least include a diagnostic hysteroscopy, saline infusion sonography, or 3D ultrasound, as 2D TVUS is not accurate enough to evaluate the precise location, number, and size of fibroids.

Despite these shortcomings in the overall body of evidence, it does seem that submucosal and cavity-distorting fibroids are associated with RPL, and that myomectomy, hysteroscopic, laparoscopic, or abdominal, is of benefit in reducing the rate of miscarriage. The benefit of surgical treatment for non-cavity-distorting fibroids is yet to be established, and subserosal and pedunculated fibroids should not be thought of as a cause of RPL. Less-invasive treatments such as medical therapy, uterine artery embolization, MRgFUS and ultrasound-guided RFA should not be offered as treatment for fibroids to women with RPL as the literature is too scant to suggest safety and efficacy of treatment in this population.

REFERENCES

1. Borgfeldt C and Andolf E. Transvaginal ultrasonographic findings in the uterus and the endometrium: Low prevalence of leiomyoma in a random sample of women age 25–40 years. *Acta Obstet Gynecol Scand.* 2000;79(3):202–7.
2. Salvador E, Bienstock J, Blakemore KJ, and Pressman E. Leiomyomata uteri, genetic amniocentesis, and the risk of second-trimester spontaneous abortion. *Am J Obstet Gynecol.* 2002;186(5):913–5.
3. Klatsky PC, Tran ND, Caughey AB, and Fujimoto VY. Fibroids and reproductive outcomes: A systematic literature review from conception to delivery. *Am J Obstet Gynecol.* 2008;198(4):357–66.
4. Laughlin SK, Baird DD, Savitz DA, Herring AH, and Hartmann KE. Prevalence of uterine leiomyomas in the first trimester of pregnancy. *Obstet Gynecol.* 2009;113(3):630–5.
5. Sheiner E, Bashiri A, Levy A, Hershkovitz R, Katz M, and Mazor M. Obstetric characteristics and perinatal outcome of pregnancies with uterine leiomyomas. *J Reprod Med.* 2004;49(3):182–6.
6. Exacoustòs C and Rosati P. Ultrasound diagnosis of uterine myomas and complications in pregnancy. *Obstet Gynecol.* 1993;82(1):97–101.
7. Shavell VI, Thakur M, Sawant A et al. Adverse obstetric outcomes associated with sonographically identified large uterine fibroids. *Fertil Steril.* 2012;97(1):107–10.
8. Pritts EA, Parker WH, and Olive DL. Fibroids and infertility: An updated systematic review of the evidence. *Fertil Steril.* 2009;91(4):1215–23.
9. Bedaiwy MA, Lepik C, and Alfaraj S. Uterine fibroids and recurrent pregnancy loss. In: Moawad N (ed). *Uterine Fibroids: A Clinical Casebook.* Cham, Switzerland: Springer; 2017, pp. 311–33.
10. Saravelos SH, Yan J, Rehmani H, and Li TC. The prevalence and impact of fibroids and their treatment on the outcome of pregnancy in women with recurrent miscarriage. *Hum Reprod.* 2011;26(12):3274–9.
11. Christiansen OB, Andersen A-MN, Bosch E et al. Evidence-based investigations and treatments of recurrent pregnancy loss. *Fertil Steril.* 2005;83(4):821–39.
12. Benson CB, Chow JS, Chang Lee W, Hill JA, and Doubilet PM. Outcome of pregnancies in women with uterine leiomyomas identified by sonography in the first trimester. *J Clin Ultrasound.* 2001;29(5):261–4.
13. Buttram VC, and Reiter RC. Uterine leiomyomata: Etiology, symptomatology, and management. *Fertil Steril.* 1981;36(4):433–45.
14. Oliveira FG, Abdelmassih VG, Diamond MP, Dozortsev D, Melo NR, and Abdelmassih R. Impact of subserosal and intramural uterine fibroids that do not distort the endometrial cavity on the outcome of *in vitro* fertilization—Intracytoplasmic sperm injection. *Fertil Steril.* 2004;81(3):582–7.
15. Sundermann AC, Velez Edwards DR, Bray MJ, Jones SH, Latham SM, and Hartmann KE. Leiomyomas in Pregnancy and Spontaneous Abortion. *Obstet Gynecol.* 2017;130(5):1065–72.
16. Ventolini G, Zhang M, and Gruber J. Hysteroscopy in the evaluation of patients with recurrent pregnancy loss: A cohort study in a primary care population. *Surg Endosc Other Interv Tech.* 2004;18(12):1782–4.
17. Cogendez E, Dolgun ZN, Sanverdi I, Turgut A, and Eren S. Post-abortion hysteroscopy: A method for early diagnosis of congenital and acquired intrauterine causes of abortions. *Eur J Obstet Gynecol Reprod Biol.* 2011;156(1):101–4.
18. Russo M, Suen M, Bedaiwy M, and Chen I. Prevalence of uterine myomas among women with 2 or more recurrent pregnancy losses: A systematic review. *J Minim Invasive Gynecol.* 2016;23(5):702–6.
19. McCormack CD, Furness DL, Dekker GA, Shand K, and Roberts CT. 3D ultrasound findings in women attending a South Australian recurrent miscarriage clinic. *Australas J Ultrasound Med.* 2016;19(4):142–6.
20. Elsokkary M, Elshourbagy M, Labib K et al. Assessment of hysteroscopic role in management of women with recurrent pregnancy loss. *J Matern Neonatal Med.* 2018;31(11):1494–504.
21. Practice Committee of the American Society for Reproductive Medicine. Evaluation and treatment of recurrent pregnancy loss: A committee opinion. *Fertil Steril.* 2012;98(5):1103–11.
22. Bohlmann MK, von Wolff M, Luedders DW et al. Hysteroscopic findings in women with two and with more than two first-trimester miscarriages are not significantly different. *Reprod Biomed Online.* 2010;21(2):230–6.

23. Seckin B, Sarikaya E, Oruc AS, Celen S, and Cicek N. Office hysteroscopic findings in patients with two, three, and four or more, consecutive miscarriages. *Eur J Contracept Reprod Heal Care*. 2012;17(5):393–8.

24. Dueholm M, Lundorf E, Hansen ES, Ledertoug S, and Olesen F. Evaluation of the uterine cavity with magnetic resonance imaging, transvaginal sonography, hysterosonographic examination, and diagnostic hysteroscopy. *Fertil Steril*. 2001;76(2):350–7.

25. Dueholm M, Lundorf E, Hansen ES, Ledertoug S, and Olesen F. Accuracy of magnetic resonance imaging and transvaginal ultrasonography in the diagnosis, mapping, and measurement of uterine myomas. *Am J Obstet Gynecol*. 2002;186(3):409–15.

26. Saravelos SH, Cocksedge KA, and Li TC. Prevalence and diagnosis of congenital uterine anomalies in women with reproductive failure: A critical appraisal. *Hum Reprod Update*. 2008;14(5):415–29.

27. Shwayder J and Sakhel K. Imaging for uterine myomas and adenomyosis. *J Minim Invasive Gynecol*. 2014;21(3):362–76.

28. Apirakviriya C, Rungruxsirivorn T, Phupong V, and Wisawasukmongchol W. Diagnostic accuracy of 3D-transvaginal ultrasound in detecting uterine cavity abnormalities in infertile patients as compared with hysteroscopy. *Eur J Obstet Gynecol Reprod Biol*. 2016;200:24–8.

29. Soares SR, Dos Reis MMBB, and Camargos AF. Diagnostic accuracy of sonohysterography, transvaginal sonography, and hysterosalpingography in patients with uterine cavity diseases. *Fertil Steril*. 2000;73(2):406–11.

30. Kubik-Huch RA, Weston M, Nougaret S et al. European Society of Urogenital Radiology (ESUR) guidelines: MR imaging of leiomyomas. *Eur Radiol*. 2018;28(8):3125–37.

31. Kaiser J and Branch DW. Recurrent pregnancy loss: Generally accepted causes and their management. *Clin Obstet Gynecol*. 2016;59(3):464–73.

32. Bailey AP, Jaslow CR, and Kutteh WH. Minimally invasive surgical options for congenital and acquired uterine factors associated with recurrent pregnancy loss. *Women's Health*. 2015;11(2):161–7.

33. De Gasperis-Brigante C, Singh SS, Vilos G, Kives S, and Murji A. Pregnancy outcomes following ulipristal acetate for uterine fibroids: A systematic review. *J Obstet Gynaecol Canada*. 2018;40(8):1066–76.e2.

34. Gingold JA, Gueye NA, and Falcone T. Minimally invasive approaches to myoma management. *J Minim Invasive Gynecol*. 2018;25(2):237–50. https://doi.org/10.1016/j.jmig.2017.07.007

35. Mashiach R, Inbar Y, Rabinovici J, Mohr Sasson A, Alagem-Mizrachi A, and Machtinger R. Outcome of magnetic resonance–guided focused ultrasound surgery (MRgFUS) for FIGO class 1 fibroids. *Eur J Obstet Gynecol Reprod Biol*. 2018;221:119–22.

36. Clark NA, Mumford SL, and Segars JH. Reproductive impact of MRI-guided focused ultrasound surgery for fibroids. *Curr Opin Obstet Gynecol*. 2014;26(3):151–61.

37. Toub DB. A new paradigm for uterine fibroid treatment: Transcervical, intrauterine sonography-guided radiofrequency ablation of uterine fibroids with the Sonata system. *Curr Obstet Gynecol Rep*. 2017;6(1):67–73.

38. Zou M, Chen L, Wu C, Hu C, and Xiong Y. Pregnancy outcomes in patients with uterine fibroids treated with ultrasound-guided high-intensity focused ultrasound. *BJOG*. 2017;124:30–5.

39. Shokeir TA. Hysteroscopic management in submuous fibroids to improve fertility. *Arch Gynecol Obstet*. 2005;273(1):50–4.

40. Roy KK, Singla S, Baruah J, Sharma JB, Kumar S, and Singh N. Reproductive outcome following hysteroscopic myomectomy in patients with infertility and recurrent abortions. *Arch Gynecol Obstet*. 2010;282(5):553–60.

41. Campo S, Campo V, and Gambadauro P. Reproductive outcome before and after laparoscopic or abdominal myomectomy for subserous or intramural myomas. *Eur J Obstet Gynecol Reprod Biol*. 2003;110(2):215–9.

42. Bernardi TS, Radosa MP, Weisheit A et al. Laparoscopic myomectomy: A 6-year follow-up single-center cohort analysis of fertility and obstetric outcome measures. *Arch Gynecol Obstet*. 2014;290(1):87–91.

43. Marchionni M, Fambrini M, Zambelli V, Scarselli G, and Susini T. Reproductive performance before and after abdominal myomectomy: A retrospective analysis. *Fertil Steril*. 2004;82(1):154–9.

44. Vercellini P, Maddalena S, De Giorgi O, Pesole A, Ferrari L, and Crosignani PG. Determinants of reproductive outcome after abdominal myomectomy for infertility. *Fertil Steril*. 1999;72(1):109–14.

45. Casini ML, Rossi F, Agostini R, and Unfer V. Effects of the position of fibroids on fertility. *Gynecol Endocrinol*. 2006;22(2):106–9.

46. Bean EMR, Cutner A, Holland T, Vashisht A, Jurkovic D, and Saridogan E. Laparoscopic myomectomy: A single-center retrospective review of 514 patients. *J Minim Invasive Gynecol.* 2017;24(3):485–93.
47. Buckley VA, Nesbitt-Hawes EM, Atkinson P et al. Laparoscopic myomectomy: Clinical outcomes and comparative evidence. *J Minim Invasive Gynecol.* 2015;22(1):11–25.
48. Tulandi T, Murray C, and Guralnick M. Adhesion formation and reproductive outcome after myomectomy and second-look laparoscopy. *Obstet Gynecol.* 1993;82(2):213–5.
49. Tulandi T, Closon F, Czuzoj-Shulman N, and Abenhaim H. Adhesion barrier use after myomectomy and hysterectomy. *Obstet Gynecol.* 2016;127(1):23–8.
50. Munro MG, Critchley HOD, Broder MS, and Fraser IS. FIGO classification system (PALM-COEIN) for causes of abnormal uterine bleeding in nongravid women of reproductive age. *Int J Gynecol Obstet.* 2011;113(1):3–13.

5

Fibroids in Pregnancy

Magdi Hanafi

CONTENTS

Introduction

Uterine fibroids (leiomyomata, myomas) are benign smooth muscle tumors of the uterus. Uterine leiomyomas/fibroids are the most common pelvic tumors of the female genital tract. The initiators remaining unknown, and estrogens and progesterone are considered as promoters of fibroid growth. Fibroids are monoclonal tumors showing 40%–50% karyotypically detectable chromosomal abnormalities. Cytogenetic aberrations involving chromosomes 6, 7, 12, and 14 constitute the major chromosome abnormalities seen in leiomyomata [1]. The potential effects of fibroids on pregnancy and the potential effects of pregnancy on fibroids are frequent clinical concerns, since these tumors are common in women of reproductive age. Most pregnant women with fibroids do not have any complications during pregnancy related to the fibroids. Pain is the most common problem, and there may be a slightly increased risk of obstetrical complications such as miscarriage, premature labor and delivery, abnormal fetal position, and placental abruption. Several factors make it difficult to assess the impact of fibroids on pregnancy outcome and to identify specific fibroid characteristics that are important.

Prevalence

The prevalence of uterine fibroids in pregnancy varies between 1.6% and 10.7%, depending on the trimester of assessment and the size threshold [2].

The prevalence of fibroids increases with age and is higher in African American women than in white or Hispanic women [3]. Increasing parity and prolonged duration of breastfeeding are associated with a small, but statistically significant, reduction in prevalence [4].

Changes in Size during Pregnancy and Postpartum

Pregnancy-related increases in estrogen and progesterone levels, uterine blood flow, and possibly human chorionic gonadotropin levels, are believed to affect fibroid growth. Most studies that have sonographically monitored the size of fibroids across pregnancy have refuted the commonly held belief that fibroids increase in size throughout gestation [5]. It appears that fibroid size remains stable (less than 10% change) across gestation in 50%–60% of cases, increases in 22%–32%, and decreases in 8%–27% [5].

Inconsistent data on the effect of pregnancy on fibroid growth may be due to the gestational age of the ultrasound assessments, since the pattern of fibroid growth during pregnancy is probably not linear [5].

For example, in those fibroids that increase in size, most of the growth occurs in the first trimester, with little if any further increase in size during the second and third trimesters [6,7]. Larger fibroids (greater than 5 cm in diameter) are more likely to grow, whereas smaller fibroids are more likely to remain stable in size [4]. The mean increase in fibroid volume during pregnancy is 12%, and very few fibroids increase by more than 25% [6,7].

Almost 90% of women with fibroids detected in the first trimester will have regression in total fibroid volume when reevaluated 3–6 months' postpartum, but 10% will have an increase in volume [8]. Regression may be less in women who use progestin-only contraception.

Symptoms

Uterine fibroids are usually asymptomatic during pregnancy (Figures 5.1 and 5.2). In symptomatic women, symptoms include pain, pelvic pressure, and/or vaginal bleeding.

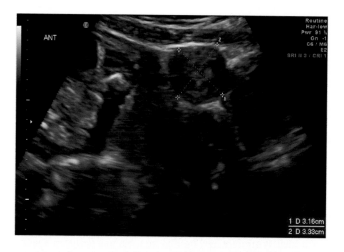

FIGURE 5.1   Fibroid compressed by the fetus. (Courtesy of Botros Rizk, Candice Holiday, and Vicki Arguello.)

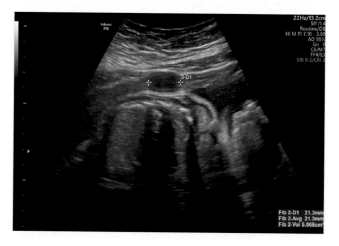

FIGURE 5.2   Fibroid in pregnancy at 27 weeks. (Courtesy of Botros Rizk, Candice Holiday, and Vicki Arguello.)

Pain is the most common symptom; the frequency correlates with size and is especially high in women with fibroids greater than 5 cm in diameter [9]. Most patients have only localized pain, without other signs and symptoms, although mild leukocytosis, fever, and nausea and vomiting can occur [10,11]. Fibroid pain typically presents in the late first or early second trimester, which corresponds to the period of greatest fibroid growth and, in turn, propensity to degeneration. Pain also may result from partial obstruction of the vessels supplying the fibroid as the uterus grows and changes its orientation to the fibroid [12], or from torsion.

Symptoms resulting from ectopic hormone production (e.g., erythropoietin, prolactin) are rare.

Complications

Uterine fibroids have long been implicated as a cause of adverse pregnancy events [13]. However, there are no well-designed studies that provide high-quality data on the relationship between fibroids and pregnancy outcome.

Most pregnant women with fibroids do not have any complications during pregnancy related to the fibroids [14]. When complications occur, painful red degeneration is the most common complication. There also appears to be a slightly increased risk of complications such as miscarriage, premature labor and delivery, abnormal fetal positions, and placental abruption, but all studies do not show an increased risk of adverse events.

Degeneration and torsion. As discussed earlier, pain is one of the most common symptoms of fibroids in pregnant women and is typically due to fibroid degeneration or, rarely, torsion. Rapid growth of fibroids can result in a relative decrease in perfusion, leading to ischemia and necrosis (red degeneration) and release of prostaglandins [15]. Pedunculated fibroids are at risk of torsion and necrosis, but this is much less common than degeneration.

Miscarriage. In some patients, submucosal fibroids appear to adversely affect implantation, placentation, and ongoing pregnancy. The effects of intramural fibroids are more controversial, while fibroids that are primarily subserosal or pedunculated are unlikely to cause adverse outcomes. The risk of pregnancy loss may be higher when there are multiple fibroids [16]. The mechanisms by which fibroids may cause pregnancy loss are not known; however, the following hypotheses have been proposed:

- The fibroid may interfere with placentation and development of normal uteroplacental circulation [17]. As an example, a large submucosal fibroid projecting into the uterine cavity may compress the decidualized endometrium, leading to decidual atrophy or distortion of the vascular architecture and blood flow supplying and draining the decidua at that site.
- Rapid fibroid growth with or without degeneration may lead to increased uterine contractility or altered production of catalytic enzymes by the placenta [17], both of which may disrupt placentation, leading to spontaneous abortion.

Preterm labor and birth. There appears to be a small increase in preterm labor and preterm birth [18] in pregnancies with uterine fibroids. Characteristics reported to increase this risk include multiple fibroids, placentation adjacent to or overlying the fibroid [5], and size greater than 5 cm.

Various theories have been proposed to explain the biologic basis of preterm labor in the setting of uterine fibroids. As an example, it is possible that fibroid uteri are less distensible than nonfibrotic uteri, so that contractions occur when the uterus distends beyond a certain point [19]. Others have noted decreased oxytocinase activity in the gravid fibroid uterus, which may result in a localized increase in oxytocin levels, thereby predisposing to premature contractions [20].

Antepartum bleeding and placental abruption. Numerous studies have reported that antepartum bleeding is more common in pregnancies with fibroids [21]. The location of the fibroid in relation to the placenta appears to be an important determinant and implies that bleeding is related to abruption.

Submucosal and retroplacental fibroids and fibroids with volumes greater than 200 mL (corresponding to 7–8 cm diameter) are associated with the highest risk of abruption [9]. As an example, in a retrospective analysis of 6706 consecutive pregnant patients, 8 out of 14 patients (57%) with retroplacental fibroids developed placental abruption with the deaths of four fetuses, while only two abruptions occurred among the 79 patients (2.5%) whose fibroids were not retroplacental, and neither of these resulted in fetal death [19].

A hypothesis for the increased risk of abruption in women with fibroids is that the fibroid causes abnormal perfusion of the placental site [19].

Malpresentation. Uterine anomalies are associated with an increased risk of malpresentation, presumably because they distort the shape of the uterine cavity [22]. One of the largest studies used a population-based cohort of over 72,000 consecutive women with singleton pregnancies in Washington State (1990–2007) who underwent routine second-trimester fetal anatomic survey at a single university hospital [23]. This study reported a significant increase in breech presentation in women with fibroids (odds ratio [OR] 1.5, 95% confidence interval [CI] 1.3–1.9). Other studies noted an increased incidence of malpresentation only if the uterus had multiple fibroids, if there was a fibroid located behind the placenta or in the lower uterine segment, or if the fibroid was large (over 10 cm) [2] (Figure 5.3).

Dysfunctional labor. Theoretically, fibroids in the myometrium may decrease the force of uterine contractions or disrupt the coordinated spread of the contractile wave, thereby leading to dysfunctional labor [24]. Several studies have reported an increased incidence of dysfunctional labor in pregnancies complicated by fibroids [24]; not all investigators have been able to confirm this association [2].

Cesarean delivery. Studies have consistently reported that uterine fibroids are associated with an increased risk of cesarean delivery [18], especially when the fibroids are located in the lower uterine segment. The proposed increase in cesarean delivery rate is likely due to such factors as an increased risk of malpresentation, dysfunctional labor, obstruction, and placental abruption.

Postpartum hemorrhage. Several studies have reported an increased risk of postpartum hemorrhage in pregnancies complicated by fibroids [2], especially if the fibroids are large (greater than 3 cm) and located behind the placenta [21] or the delivery is by cesarean [26]. Numerous other studies have found no association between fibroids and postpartum hemorrhage [5]. Pathophysiologically, fibroids could predispose to postpartum hemorrhage by decreasing both the force and coordination of uterine contractions, thereby leading to uterine atony [27].

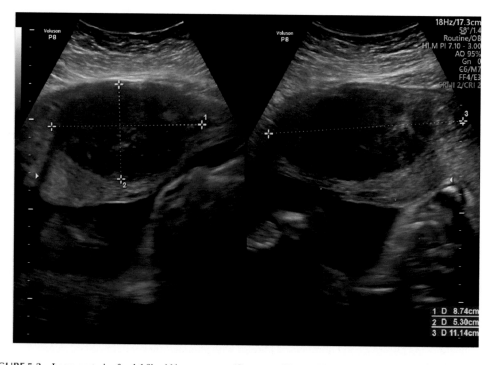

FIGURE 5.3   Large posterior fundal fibroid in pregnancy. (Courtesy of Botros Rizk, Candice Holiday, and Vicki Arguello.)

Fetal anomalies. Spatial restrictions from uterine fibroids can cause fetal deformations, but this is extremely rare. Case reports have described fetal anomalies including limb reduction defects, congenital torticollis, and head deformities in pregnancies with large submucosal fibroids [28].

Preterm premature rupture of membranes. Pooled cumulative data suggest that fibroids do not increase the risk of premature rupture of membranes and may even slightly decrease the risk [18]. However, individual studies have reported conflicting findings [2,9,21,23]. The location of the fibroid in relation to the placenta may be an important determinant: the greatest risk of preterm premature rupture of membranes appears to be when the fibroid is in direct contact with the placenta [21].

Placenta previa. Most studies that account for maternal age and prior uterine surgery failed to show any association between fibroids and placenta previa [5], although two large series reported an increased rate (1.4% versus 0.5% in controls [23], 3.8% versus 2% in controls [2]). The latter series adjusted for prior cesarean delivery and myomectomy.

Fetal growth restriction. Fibroids have minimal, if any, effect on fetal growth. It is possible, however, that large fibroids (greater than 200 mL) may be associated with delivery of small-for-gestational age infants (less than the 10th percentile for gestational age) [7].

Other complications. A number of other pregnancy complications have been reported in women with fibroids, including disseminated intravascular coagulation, spontaneous hemoperitoneum, uterine incarceration, urinary tract obstruction with urinary retention or acute renal failure, deep vein thrombosis, and puerperal uterine inversion [29].

Pyomyoma (suppurative leiomyoma) is rare [30]. Clinical findings may include fever, leukocytosis, tachycardia, pelvic pain, and characteristic features on imaging studies (heterogeneous mass that may contain gas).

Fetal demise. Rates of intrauterine fetal demise are not increased in pregnancies complicated by uterine fibroids [31].

Preeclampsia. The majority of studies do not support an association between fibroids and preeclampsia, although one study noted that women with multiple fibroids were significantly more likely to develop preeclampsia than those with a single fibroid (45% versus 13%) [32]. The increased risk was due to disruption of trophoblast invasion by the multiple fibroids leading to inadequate uteroplacental vascular remodeling leading to the development of preeclampsia.

Management Issues

Indications for preconception myomectomy decisions are made on a case-by-case basis and depend on age, past reproductive history, severity of symptoms, and size and location of the fibroids.

Myomectomy during pregnancy or at delivery is potentially harmful (hemorrhage, uterine rupture, miscarriage, or preterm delivery). Myomectomy should be avoided during pregnancy and at delivery, especially if an intramyometrial incision is required, unless the procedure cannot be safely delayed [9,10,15]. Uncontrollable hemorrhage during myomectomy may necessitate hysterectomy.

Rarely, myomectomy of pedunculated or subserosal fibroids has been performed antepartum for management of an acute abdomen or obstruction, and myomectomy may be required at cesarean delivery in order to close the hysterotomy.

Painful fibroids. Pregnant women with painful fibroids may require hospitalization for pain management [9]. We suggest supportive care and administration of acetaminophen as the initial intervention.

Short-term use of opioids in standard doses or a course of nonsteroidal anti-inflammatory drugs (NSAIDs) can be given when pain is not controlled by these measures. First-trimester opioid use has been associated with an increased risk of congenital anomalies in some studies, but the data are weak and do not justify withholding these medications when needed to control pain.

Pain may be managed with a short course of ibuprofen [10]. Indomethacin 25 mg orally every 6 hours for up to 48 hours is another NSAID that has been effective [11]. Therapy should be limited to pregnancies less than 32 weeks of gestation because of the possibility of inducing premature closure of the ductus arteriosus, neonatal pulmonary hypertension, oligohydramnios, and fetal/neonatal platelet dysfunction [11]. If indomethacin is continued for more than 48 hours, weekly sonographic assessment for oligohydramnios and narrowing of the fetal ductus arteriosus should be performed. If either of these findings is noted, indomethacin should either be discontinued or reduced to 25 mg every 12 hours. Repeat courses can be given as needed for recurrent episodes of pain. Although first-trimester use of NSAIDs has been associated with miscarriage in some studies, the best data do not support an association [33]. The use of a local protected heating pad may be safer for the pregnancy if the patient tolerates its use and is less ambulatory.

Case reports have described successful use of epidural analgesia for treatment of severe pain refractory to other therapies [34].

Fibroids prolapsing into the vagina. Elective removal of prolapsed fibroids in pregnancy is generally advised against as the risks likely outweigh the benefits, unless there is an easily accessible pedunculated fibroid on a thin stalk. Removal may lead to hemorrhage, rupture of membranes, and/or pregnancy loss.

The need for resection should be assessed on a case-by-case basis. Clinically significant bleeding, excessive pain, urinary retention, and (rarely) infection during pregnancy due to a prolapsed fibroid are reasonable indications for resection. Symptomatic fibroids in pregnant women have been successfully removed transvaginally [35]. The procedure for transvaginal myomectomy depends on the origin of the fibroid (cervix versus submucosa) and thickness of the stalk/base, which can be determined clinically or by transvaginal ultrasound or magnetic resonance imaging (MRI), if necessary. An asymptomatic lower uterine segment submucosal prolapsed fibroid may become intrauterine with advancing gestation with partial or total nonvisualization of the prolapsed fibroid tumor vaginally.

Route of delivery. Most patients with fibroids will have a successful vaginal delivery and thus should be offered a trial of labor. Cesarean delivery is reserved for standard obstetrical indications (e.g., malpresentation, failure to progress). Elective cesarean delivery may be considered because of concerns that fetal descent will be obstructed, but it should be limited to women most likely to fail a trial of labor, including those with large cervical fibroids or with lower uterine segment fibroids that distort the uterine cavity and are located between the fetal vertex and cervix in the third trimester [36].

Operative issues at cesarean delivery. A third-trimester hemoglobin level of at least 9.5–10 mg/dL or above is desirable in women at high risk of intrapartum or postpartum hemorrhage at the time of cesarean delivery, such as women with large, retroplacental or anterior lower uterine segment fibroids; use of a cell saver and availability of blood products in a cooler should be considered on a case-by-case basis.

A vertical skin incision and a posterior or classical hysterotomy are sometimes necessary to obtain adequate exposure when the fibroids are located in the lower uterine segment. Every effort should be made to avoid transecting a fibroid during hysterotomy, as the incision may be impossible to close without first removing the tumor, which can cause excessive uterine wall bleeding. A limited elective myomectomy at cesarean delivery may be possible for patients with symptomatic pedunculated fibroids, which is more likely in pregnant women since the term uterus receives 17% of cardiac output [37]. In a case series of nine patients who underwent myomectomy at the time of cesarean delivery, three (33%) were complicated by severe hemorrhage requiring puerperal hysterectomy [9].

Other interventions to minimize maternal morbidity are under investigation. In a pilot study, uterine artery ligation at the time of cesarean delivery appeared to enhance shrinkage of fibroids postpartum [38], but further clinical studies and risk/benefit analyses are needed before such an intervention can be recommended.

Management of Patients with Prior Myomectomy

Method of delivery and timing of cesarean delivery. In the absence of strong evidence of the absolute risk of rupture, it is recommended to take a conservative approach and perform cesarean delivery prior to the onset of labor if the myometrium was significantly compromised by previous surgery, such as entry into the uterine cavity or near entry during a prior myomectomy or if a large number of myomas were removed. Committee opinion by the American College of Obstetricians and Gynecologists (ACOG) recommends that women with previous myomectomy undergo cesarean delivery between 370/7th and 386/7th weeks of gestation, although consideration of delivery as early as 36 weeks is reasonable for women with prior extensive myomectomy (analogous to a patient with prior classical hysterotomy) [39].

For patients who have had an intramyometrial myomectomy that was unlikely to have significantly compromised the myometrium, it is recommended to have a trial of labor with continuous intrapartum fetal monitoring, early access to obstetric anesthesia, and the ability to perform an emergency cesarean delivery, as needed. Patients who have had a pedunculated fibroid removed would not be expected to have compromised the integrity of the myometrium and do not require special monitoring during labor.

The magnitude of the risk of uterine rupture in pregnancies after myomectomy and specific criteria associated with increased risk are difficult to ascertain because of the small number of cases reported and lack of detail about the operative procedures performed. Available data, although limited, suggest that the risk of uterine rupture after myomectomy is not significantly greater than that for a patient attempting trial of labor after cesarean. In a 2016 systematic review of studies with at least five cases of pregnancy after myomectomy, the overall incidence of uterine rupture after myomectomy was 7/756 or 0.93% (95% CI 0.45%–1.92%) [40]. The incidence was 0.47% (2/426, 95% CI 0.13%–1.70%) in women undergoing trial of labor after myomectomy and 1.52% (5/330%, 95% CI 0.65%–3.51%) in women before the onset of labor; this difference was not statistically significant. Six of the seven ruptures occurred in women who had a prior laparoscopic myomectomy, which has been attributed to the technical challenge of laparoscopic suturing [41]. All ruptures occurred following myomectomy of an intramural fibroid, although this was not noted to be a significant risk factor for uterine rupture. The uterine cavity was not entered during myomectomy in three cases; this information was not available in the other four cases. The ruptures occurred at 24 (twins), 25, 30, 32, 36, 37, and 40 weeks of gestation; however, this finding may be biased by scheduled cesarean deliveries at term.

It is important for the gynecologist who performs any type of myomectomy to clearly identify in the operative note the number, size, and location of the tumor; the depth and number of uterine incisions; and any entrance of the uterine cavity. A recommendation to the future obstetrician of whether elective cesarean section or trial of labor for the possible coming pregnancies is advisable. This recommendation must be stated clearly to the patient and noted in the patient's records.

Abnormal placentation. Prior hysteroscopic myomectomy of a submucosal fibroid may increase the risk of abnormal placentation, especially placenta accreta due to the increased chance of adhesion formation in the uterine cavity. Although the risk of placenta accreta after prior myomectomy appears to be low [25], data are sparse. Ultrasound screening for possible placenta accreta in the late second or early third trimester is recommended.

REFERENCES

1. Medikare V, Kandukuri LR, Ananthapur V, Deenadayal M, and Nallari P. The genetic bases of uterine fibroids: A review. *J Reprod Infertil*. 2011;12(3):181–91.
2. Qidwai GI, Caughey AB, and Jacoby AF. Obstetric outcomes in women with sonographically identified uterine leiomyomata. *Obstet Gynecol*. 2006;107:376.
3. Laughlin SK, Baird DD, Savitz DA et al. Prevalence of uterine leiomyomas in the first trimester of pregnancy: An ultrasound-screening study. *Obstet Gynecol*. 2009;113:630.
4. Terry KL, De Vivo I, Hankinson SE, and Missmer SA. Reproductive characteristics and risk of uterine leiomyomata. *Fertil Steril*. 2010;94:2703.
5. Lev-Toaff AS, Coleman BG, Arger PH et al. Leiomyomas in pregnancy: Sonographic study. *Radiology*. 1987;164:375.
6. Aharoni A, Reiter A, Golan D et al. Patterns of growth of uterine leiomyomas during pregnancy. A prospective longitudinal study. *Br J Obstet Gynaecol*. 1988;95:510.
7. Rosati P, Exacoustòs C, and Mancuso S. Longitudinal evaluation of uterine myoma growth during pregnancy. A sonographic study. *J Ultrasound Med*. 1992;11:511.
8. Laughlin SK, Hartmann KE, and Baird DD. Postpartum factors and natural fibroid regression. *Am J Obstet Gynecol*. 2011;204:496.el.
9. Exacoustòs C and Rosati P. Ultrasound diagnosis of uterine myomas and complications in pregnancy. *Obstet Gynecol*. 1993;82:97.
10. Katz VL, Dotters DJ, and Droegemeuller W. Complications of uterine leiomyomas in pregnancy. *Obstet Gynecol*. 1989;73:593.

11. Dildy GA 3rd, Moise KJ Jr, Smith LG Jr et al. Indomethacin for the treatment of symptomatic leiomyoma uteri during pregnancy. *Am J Perinatol.* 1992;9:185.

12. Parker WH. Etiology, symptomatology, and diagnosis of uterine myomas. *Fertil Steril.* 2007;87:725.

13. Lynch FW. Fibroid tumors complicating pregnancy and labor. *Am J Obstet.* 1913;68:427.

14. Segars JH, Parrott EC, Nagel JD et al. Proceedings from the Third National Institutes of Health International Congress on Advances in Uterine Leiomyoma Research: Comprehensive review, conference summary and future recommendations. *Hum Reprod Update.* 2014;20:309.

15. De Carolis S, Fatigante G, Ferrazzani S et al. Uterine myomectomy in pregnant women. *Fetal Diagn Ther.* 2001;16:116.

16. Benson CB, Chow JS, Chang-Lee W et al. Outcome of pregnancies in women with uterine leiomyomas identified by sonography in the first trimester. *J Clin Ultrasound.* 2001;29:261.

17. Wallach EE and Vu KK. Myomata uteri and infertility. *Obstet Gynecol Clin North Am.* 1995;22:791.

18. Klatsky PC, Tran ND, Caughey AB, and Fujimoto VY. Fibroids and reproductive outcomes: A systematic literature review from conception to delivery. *Am J Obstet Gynecol.* 2008;198:357.

19. Rice JP, Kay HH, and Mahony BS. The clinical significance of uterine leiomyomas in pregnancy. *Am J Obstet Gynecol.* 1989;160:1212.

20. Blum M. Comparative study of serum CAP activity during pregnancy in malformed and normal uterus. *J Perinat Med.* 1978;6:165.

21. Muram D, Gillieson M, and Walters JH. Myomas of the uterus in pregnancy: Ultrasonographic follow-up. *Am J Obstet Gynecol.* 1980;138:16.

22. Heinonen PK, Saarikoski S, and Pystynen P. Reproductive performance of women with uterine anomalies. An evaluation of 182 cases. *Acta Obstet Gynecol Scand.* 1982;61:157.

23. Stout MJ, Odibo AO, Graseck AS et al. Leiomyomas at routine second-trimester ultrasound examination and adverse obstetric outcomes. *Obstet Gynecol.* 2010;116:1056.

24. Vergani P, Ghidini A, Strobelt N et al. Do uterine leiomyomas influence pregnancy outcome? *Am J Perinatol.* 1994;11:356.

25. Gyamfi-Bannerman C, Gilbert S, Landon MB et al. Risk of uterine rupture and placenta accreta with prior uterine surgery outside of the lower segment. *Obstet Gynecol.* 2012;120:1332.

26. Hasan F, Arumugam K, and Sivanesaratnam V. Uterine leiomyomata in pregnancy. *Int J Gynaecol Obstet.* 1991;34:45.

27. Szamatowicz J, Laudanski T, Bulkszas B, and Akerlund M. Fibromyomas and uterine contractions. *Acta Obstet Gynecol Scand.* 1997;76:973.

28. Graham JM, Miller ME, Stephan MJ, and Smith DW. Limb reduction anomalies and early in utero limb compression. *J Pediatr.* 1980;96:1052.

29. Phelan JP. Myomas and pregnancy. *Obstet Gynecol Clin North Am.* 1995;22:801.

30. Laubach M, Breugelmans M, Leyder M et al. Nonsurgical treatment of pyomyoma in the postpartum period. *Surg Infect (Larchmt).* 2011;12:65.

31. Koike T, Minakami H, Kosuge S et al. Uterine leiomyoma in pregnancy: Its influence on obstetric performance. *J Obstet Gynaecol Res.* 1999;25:309.

32. Roberts WE, Fulp KS, Morrison JC, and Martin JN Jr. The impact of leiomyomas on pregnancy. *Aust N Z J Obstet Gynaecol.* 1999;39:43.

33. Daniel S, Koren G, Lunenfeld E et al. Fetal exposure to nonsteroidal anti-inflammatory drugs and spontaneous abortions. *CMAJ.* 2014;186:E177.

34. Treissman DA, Bate JT, and Randall PT. Epidural use of morphine in managing the pain of carneous degeneration of a uterine leiomyoma during pregnancy. *Can Med Assoc J.* 1982;126:505.

35. Kilpatrick CC, Adler MT, and Chohan L. Vaginal myomectomy in pregnancy: A report of two cases. *South Med J.* 2010;103:1058.

36. Tian J, and Hu W. Cervical leiomyomas in pregnancy: Report of 17 cases. *Aust N Z J Obstet Gynaecol.* 2012;52:258.

37. Gabbe SG, Niebyl JR, and Simpson JL. *Obstetrics: Normal and Problem Pregnancies.* 4th ed. Philadelphia, PA: Churchill Livingstone, 2008, p. 739.

38. Liu WM, Wang PH, Tang WL et al. Uterine artery ligation for treatment of pregnant women with uterine leiomyomas who are undergoing cesarean section. *Fertil Steril.* 2006;86:423.

39. American College of Obstetricians and Gynecologists. ACOG committee opinion no. 560: Medically indicated late-preterm and early-term deliveries. *Obstet Gynecol.* 2013;121:908.

40. Gambacorti-Passerini Z, Gimovsky AC, Locatelli A, and Berghella V. Trial of labor after myomectomy and uterine rupture: A systematic review. *Acta Obstet Gynecol Scand.* 2016;95:724.

41. Nezhat C. The "cons" of laparoscopic myomectomy in women who may reproduce in the future. *Int J Fertil Menopausal Stud.* 1996;41:280.

6

Medical Options for Uterine Fibroids in the Context of Reproduction

Hoda Elkafas, Mona Al Helou, Qiwei Yang, and Ayman Al-Hendy

CONTENTS

Introduction

Uterine fibroids are the most common benign myometrial tumors affecting 70%–80% of women during their lifetime [1–3]. In the United States, the annual economic burden of these tumors is evaluated to be $34.4 billion [4]. The rate of this disease can be affected by many factors, including race, body mass index, family history, and ethnicities. Although uterine fibroids are benign tumors, they can cause heavy menstrual bleeding (HMB), pelvic pain, preterm labor, recurrent abortion, urinary incontinence, and infertility. In addition to myomectomy and hysterectomy, which are the primary surgical treatments for fibroids, the current treatment also includes gonadotropin-releasing hormone (GnRH) agonist, which decreases tumor size by 40% in 3 months. Unfortunately, GnRH agonists have limited use due to their hypoestrogenic side effects [2,5]. Uterine fibroids are monoclonal tumors that arise from uterine smooth muscle (myometrium), and one of their characteristic features is their dependency on the ovarian steroids estrogen (E2) and progesterone (P4) [6]. Hormonal fluctuations influence fibroid growth during the pregnancy and postpartum periods. In addition to the hormonal response, these lesions are influenced by genetic aberrations [7,8]. The monoclonal origin of fibroids implies mutations of myometrial cells as the origin of the disease. Clonal chromosomal aberrations are detected in approximately 20% of the fibroids. Of these, recurrent chromosomal translocations, including chromosomal regions 12q1415 or 6p21, respectively, that report for the most of cytogenetic deviations, lead to transcriptional upregulation of the human high mobility group AT-hook (HMGA) genes following by activation of the p14Arf–p53 network. It is well studied that fibroids can be subdivided based on the presence of clonal chromosomal aberrations as, e.g., deletions of the long arm of chromosome 7, trisomy 12 or chromosomal rearrangements targeting both of the two human HMGA genes [2,9,10]. Recently, research on a somatic mutation (c.131G > A) in the mediator complex subunit 12 gene (MED12) has been undertaken, as this is a primary subscriber to fibroid pathogenesis. Mutations in exon 2 of MED12 are present in approximately 85% of uterine fibroids [2]. Sex steroid hormones are also suggested to play a role in fibroid occurrence. Estrogen has a crucial role in fibroid growth and development, which explains the onset of symptoms at puberty and stops after menopause. Uterine fibroids have more estrogen and progesterone receptors than healthy myometrial cells. Progesterone's role in pathogenesis is still poorly understood, but studies showed that it affects fibroid growth. Early life exposure to endocrine-disrupting chemicals, such as diethylstilbestrol (DES), genistein, dioxin, and bisphenol-A (BPA), can change the function of the endocrine system by binding hormone receptors or by revising hormone synthesis and metabolism, leading to hyperresponsiveness to normal levels of estrogen, which increases the risk of fibroid development [11–13].

Risk Factors of Uterine Fibroids

Race

The incidence of uterine fibroids is disproportionately higher in African American women compared with Caucasian women. The prevalence of fibroids by age 50 years is higher than 80% in African American women, compared with 70% in Caucasian women. Compared to Caucasian women, African American women are 2.4- and 6.8-fold more likely to have a hysterectomy and myomectomy for treatment of fibroids, respectively. Notwithstanding the disproportionate severity and incidence of fibroids in African American women, the underlying reason for the disparity is not well known. More studies on the etiology of uterine fibroids are required to identify the reason for ethnic risk factors in fibroids [14].

Reproductive Factors

Parity and pregnancy play a protective role in uterine fibroid development, decreasing the risk of uterine fibroids up to five fold, first due to the decreased interval of exposure to unopposed estrogen and second due to the occurrence of ischemia during parturition and uterine remodeling. Breastfeeding has no effect on uterine fibroid penetrance. The underlying biological mechanisms are not well understood, but many studies of menarche showed that an increased risk of uterine fibroids is associated with earlier age [15].

Obesity

High body mass index is associated with a reasonable increase in risk of uterine fibroids. Obesity leads to an increase in the conversion of adrenal androgens to estrogen, eventually resulting in more unbound active estrogen. Also, hyperinsulinemia that leads to metabolic syndrome was found to be associated with an increased risk of uterine fibroids [16].

Vitamin D Deficiency

Vitamin D deficiency was found to increase the incidence of uterine fibroids. Reduced levels of vitamin D receptor in fibroids were associated with increased levels of ER-α, PR-A, or PR-B that would cause proliferation in myometrial cells and consequently fibroid occurrence. The presence of 1, 25 (OH)2D$_3$ may reduce estrogen-induced proliferation in myometrial cells [17,84].

Hormonal Effects

Clinical and experimental studies have shown that estrogen and progesterone stimulate the growth of uterine fibroids. A prominent feature of uterine fibroids is their dependency on the ovarian steroid hormones through the reproductive years. Regression is seen after menopause, or after treatment with gonadotropin-releasing hormone (GnRH) agonist. GnRH inhibits uterine fibroid growth by diminishing ovarian hormone production.

Estrogens, such as 17β-estradiol, exert their natural effects on target cells, including myometrial cells, through the activation of estrogen receptors (ERs), such as ERα and ER. Estrogen exhibits its action via genomic and nongenomic mechanisms [18,19].

Progesterone is an endogenous steroid hormone associated with the menstrual cycle and pregnancy and has an essential role in female reproduction and pregnancy. Like estrogen, progesterone exerts an effect by binding to the progesterone receptor (PR). There are several types of PRs, including PR-A and PR-B. The PR-B isoform is identical to PR-A but with an extra 165 amino acids. Progesterone exhibits its action via genomic and nongenomic mechanisms [20]. The capability of PR isoforms to target different promoters and control the expression of various downstream genes is influenced in a cell- and context-specific manner, including the functional interaction of PRs with other transcriptional factors [21]. In uterine fibroids, progesterone controls many targets, which may play an essential role in uterine fibroid pathogenesis [22]. A direct functional link between progesterone and uterine fibroid development was shown in a mouse xenograft model, reflecting characteristics of uterine fibroids by grafting human fibroid tissue beneath the renal capsule of immunodeficient mice. In this model, fibroid growth was induced by an administration of estrogen plus progesterone and was blocked by the PR antagonist RU486. The mass of established fibroid xenografts shows statistically significant diminishment in response to progesterone withdrawal, suggesting that the volume maintenance and growth of fibroids are progesterone dependent [6]. Antiprogestins are capable of binding to PR, which disrupts the unnecessary growth of cells giving rise to gynecological diseases, including uterine fibroids [23]. Clinical data demonstrate that although antiprogestin treatment inhibits fibroid growth, total regression of fibroids is not observed, and fibroids can reappear after treatment cessation [18].

Uterine Fibroid Management

Treatment options of uterine fibroids include medical and surgical options. Women try to avoid the surgical option due to the risks associated with the operation and to save their uterus for future pregnancies. Medical options are preferred; however, sometimes surgical intervention is considered the primary choice of treatment for uterine fibroids [24,25]. In this chapter, we cover uterine fibroid treatment options by addressing their impact on productivity maintenance.

Surgical and nonsurgical strategies include myomectomy by hysteroscopy, myomectomy done by laparotomy or laparoscopy, uterine artery embolization (UAE), and other interventions done under radiologic or ultrasound guidance [26] (Figure 6.1).

Hysteroscopic Myomectomy

Hysteroscopy is a modality by which intrauterine pathologies can be diagnosed and treated at the same time. The extraction of submucosal fibroids is one of the main indications for hysteroscopic myomectomy. Surgical resection by hysteroscopy increases pregnancy rates in submucosal fibroids, while myomectomy for intramural fibroids is still discussed. Complexities include uterine perforation that might lead to nearby organ injury, postoperative endometritis, and bleeding [24].

Laparoscopic Myomectomy

Minimally invasive laparoscopic surgery allows for less postoperative pain, a lower rate of postoperative fever, a shorter hospital stay, and a rapid recovery time with a speedier return to performance and

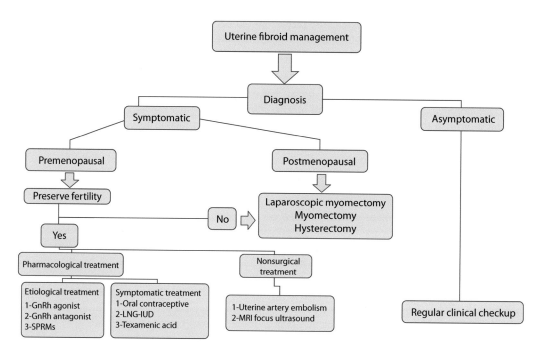

FIGURE 6.1 Uterine fibroid management.

movements of daily living, when compared with an open surgical method. Laparoscopic myomectomy is safe and efficient, with a low complication rate of less than 10%. Its pitfall might be a longer operative time [25]. Several complications have been seen in laparoscopic myomectomy, the most concerning and worrisome complication of laparoscopic myomectomy is a pregnancy-related uterine rupture. Though it comprised only a small proportion of complications, it can be lethal to both the pregnant woman and her baby when it occurs.

Uterine rupture is a fatal complication, and the risk is unpredictable. When considering laparoscopic myomectomy in reproductive-aged women, the risk should not be overlooked [26].

Uterine Artery Embolization

UAE is a radiologic intervention used when there are symptomatic fibroids. It is contraindicated in pelvic inflammatory disease, uterine malignancy, or pregnancy. Relative contraindications include severe renal insufficiency not managed by dialysis or a refractory coagulopathy. UAE has a more significant safety profile and allows for shorter hospital stays when compared to hysterectomy, as well as results in better patient satisfaction. Complications associated with UAE are postembolization syndrome that is rarely serious, endometritis, delayed contrast material reactions, tube-ovarian or uterine abscess, amenorrhea, urinary tract infection, urinary retention, fibroid sloughing requiring hysteroscopic extraction or hysterectomy, and uterine infarction [27].

Pharmacological Therapies for Uterine Fibroids

So far, therapies for fibroids are limited, and no pharmacological agent is accepted and approved for long-term treatment of fibroids [27]. The primary treatments of uterine fibroids—myomectomy and hysterectomy—have been recognized and announced as solutions for all cases. However, these options are only for women who are not planning for future pregnancies. For women who refuse surgical operation and prepare for future fertility, the best treatment choice is to control and stabilize hormone levels at uterine fibroid cells. Drug-based strategies have been traditionally accepted as a presurgical adjuvant to diminish fibroid volume, but not for long-term treatment plans. Current pharmaceuticals either fail to fix

TABLE 6.1

Recent Therapies for the Treatment and Control of Uterine Fibroids

Class	Drug Example	Mechanism of Action	Adverse Effects	U.S. FDA Approved
GnRH agonist	Leuprolide	Flare-up effect pituitary suppression	1. Decrease BMD 2. Severe vasomotor symptoms	Approved for fibroids
Progestogen	LNG-IUS	Direct release of levonorgestrel	1. Breakthrough bleeding and spotting (first 3–6 months) 2. Expulsion	Approved for HMB
Combined oral contraceptives	Estradiol valerate/ dienogest	Inhibit ovulation by downregulation of sex steroid hormones	Venous thromboembolism	Approved for HMB
GnRh antagonist	1. Elagolix (Orilissa) 2. Relugolix 3. OBE210 (ObsEva)	Short-acting, competitive antagonists of GnRH	1. Decrease BMD 2. Severe vasomotor symptoms	Approved (May 29, 2020)
SPRMs	1-Mefiprestone	First SPRM with antagonist effect	1. Decrease BMD 2. Severe vasomotor symptoms	Not approved
	2-Asoprisnil	Progesterone antagonist	Endometrial hyperplasia	Not approved
	3-Telapristone	Progesterone antagonist	PAECs	Not approved
	4-Ulipristal acetate	Mixed agonist-antagonist effects	Increase liver enzymes	Not approved
	5-Vilaprisan	Progesterone antagonist	PAECs	Not approved

Abbreviations: U.S. FDA, U.S. Food and Drug Administration; BMD, bone mineral density; GnRH, gonadotropin-releasing hormone; HMB, heavy menstrual bleeding; LNG-IUS, levonorgestrel-releasing intrauterine system; PAEC, progesterone receptor modulator associated endometrial change; SPRM, selective progesterone receptor modulator.

symptoms entirely or are correlated with unacceptable side effects that restrict their long-term use [27]. Ongoing studies in the field predict fibroid drug treatment options for a significant role beyond short-term preoperative adjuvant therapy. Unfortunately, traditional hormonal therapy carries an intrinsic side effect for a long-term treatment option. Here, we cover the main pharmacological agents that were considered or are currently being investigated for their role in uterine fibroid management, with particular stress on selective progesterone receptor modulators (SPRMs) and GnRH agonists and antagonists. The mechanism of action, side effects, and trials of modern, emerging medical options for treating and controlling the symptoms of uterine fibroids and their approval status by the U.S. Food and Drug Administration (FDA) are reviewed and summarized in Table 6.1.

Combined Oral Contraceptives

Combined oral contraceptives (COCs) are considered the first-line treatment to control abnormal uterine bleeding (AUB) without decreasing uterine fibroid size. COCs inhibit ovulation by downregulating sex steroid hormones. They are a low-cost treatment with an excellent safety profile; however, young women at risk for uterine fibroids cannot be administered COCs due to their androgenic effects and increased risk of arterial thrombosis [27,28].

Levonorgestrel-Releasing Intrauterine System

The levonorgestrel-releasing intrauterine system (LNG-IUS) was the first contraceptive method designed for long-term treatment up to 5 years. LNG-IUS works through direct release of LNG into the endometrial lining which suppresses proliferation, causing endometrial atrophy, and amenorrhea. LNG-IUS has less systemic adverse effects compared with COCs. In 2009, the FDA approved the LNG-IUS contraceptive method in the treatment of HMB, which improved quality of life with long-term treatment [28].

Progestogens

High-dose oral progestogens are the commonly prescribed treatment for short-term management of HMB in women with or without uterine fibroids [29]. In randomized controlled trials (RCTs), norethisterone (5 mg three times per day at days 5–26 of the menstrual cycle) was shown to reduce menstrual blood loss (MBL) by greater than 80 mL versus the LNG-IUS [30]. This effect is most likely due to endometrium decidualization. Based on a review of RCTs, use of progestogens in women with uterine fibroids is limited [31]. But in a study using high-dose depot medroxyprogesterone acetate (MPA) as an add-back therapy, the effects of leuprolide acetate on uterine fibroid size reduction were reversed by MPA [32], which confirms the effect of progesterone in uterine fibroid pathogenesis. But high-dose progestogens, either as a monotherapy or as an add-back therapy in combination with GnRH agonists, do not seem to be suitable for the management of symptomatic uterine fibroids because long-term treatment with progestogens is associated with increased bleeding and spotting via changes in endometrial vasculature [33].

Selective Progesterone Receptor Modulators

Estrogen was known as the primary ovarian hormone involved in uterine fibroid growth and continuance. Recent findings have recommended a more significant role of progesterone and its corresponding receptors than previously considered by providing a new target for therapy improvement [34,35]. Initially, the term *progesterone receptor modulator* (PRM) included both progesterone receptor agonist, progesterone receptor antagonist (antiprogestin), and SPRMs. SPRMS are ligands that have selective progesterone agonist, antagonist, or dual activity on various progesterone tissues [36]. Only mixed PR agonists and PR antagonists with tissue/organ selectivity were included in this category. All PRMs involved in clinical trials are 11β-benzaldoxime-substituted steroids [28].

The SPRM family includes mifepristone (the first member of this family), asoprisnil, onapristone, ulipristal acetate (UPA), lonaprisan, vilaprisan, and telapristone. These SPRMs have been investigated in clinical studies for various women's health conditions [36]. These ligands have different actions based on PR selectivity and the degree of progesterone agonist activity *in vivo* [37,38]. Those compounds have been evaluated in women with HMB and uterine fibroids [39], and SPRMs were capable of shrinking uterine fibroid volume by 17%–57% and reducing uterine mass by 9%–53% [25]. Unlike GnRH agonists, SPRMs lack the hypoestrogenic effect and the bone mineral density (BMD) loss. The recurrence of uterine fibroids is reduced up to 6 months, even by stopping treatment with SPRMs [40]. Cochrane review on SPRMs highlighted the improvement of the patient's quality of the life undergoing treatment with SPRMs for 3 months by reducing HMB, decrease uterine fibroid size and reduce the uterine volume compared with placebos group [41].

The molecular effects of modulating progesterone and its receptors are still under study, as it has been shown that progesterone has both proliferative and antiproliferative effects. Recently, it was found that the effect of SPRMs is augmented after increased expression of progesterone receptors within fibroids when compared to the adjacent myometrium [27,40]. Progesterone's effects include decreasing expression of tumor necrosis factor-alpha (TNF-α), stimulation of epidermal growth factor (EGF), and antiapoptosis. Also, it can downregulate Bcl-2 and insulin-like growth factor-1 (IGF-1) [42]. Current theories suggest that SPRMs cause apoptosis in tumor cells and downregulate the proliferation of cells involved in collagen synthesis, with subsequent extracellular matrix (ECM) reduction and fibroid shrinking [6,42] (Figure 6.2).

Mifepristone (RU-486) is one of the most common antiprogestins. It initially has antagonistic activity on PRs [43]. Several dosages of mifepristone were involved in clinical trials to examine its effects on tumor regression and symptom improvement. Regarding RU-486 dosage, lower doses of mifepristone seem to have an effect on symptoms and can diminish uterine fibroid volume, but the use of high doses has some antiglucocorticoid activity [44,45], up to 50%. A meta-analysis of 11 RCTs found that mifepristone at 2.5 mg/d for 3–6 months significantly reduced uterine and fibroid volume [46]. Mifepristone could be

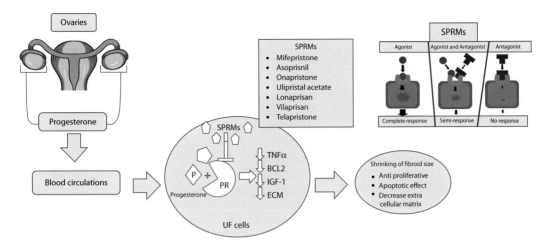

FIGURE 6.2 Role of progesterone in uterine fibroid pathogenesis. Ovarian progesterone works as an agonist at the progesterone receptor (PR), while selective progesterone receptor modulators work as antagonists at the PR and block transcription of critical genes for apoptosis, proliferation, and extracellular matrix formation.

used to shrink uterine fibroids before surgery [46]. Another meta-analysis of three RCTs on mifepristone found that it enhanced the fibroid-related quality of life (based on the uterine fibroids Symptom Quality of Life Scale) and reduced heavy bleeding symptoms, but did not significantly shrink uterine fibroid volume [41]. As such, better-controlled trials are necessary with long-term implications to assess the use of mifepristone in uterine fibroids.

UPA is a selective progesterone modulator that has been approved in the European Union and Canada for short-term therapy for symptomatic uterine fibroids. Although UPA is FDA approved as an urgency contraceptive, it has been shown to be well tolerated in premenopausal women with symptomatic fibroids [47]. It was used as a preoperative medication for symptomatic fibroids based on short-term RCTs in females with uterine fibroids associated with HMB [48,49], and recently as an alternative therapy of mild to critical symptoms of uterine fibroids in adult women of reproductive age [50]. The proper mechanisms of the PRM's action in women with HMB and fibroids are complicated and include direct effects on ovulation, endometrial vessels, uterine blood flow, and direct PR-mediated effects on uterine fibroid cells such as antiproliferative and proapoptotic effects, as well as inhibition of ECM production [51].

UPA has tissue-specific progesterone with dual agonist and antagonist effects [52]. UPA has different mechanisms to control fibroid growth on a molecular basis including promoting apoptosis in fibroid cells, downregulating vascular endothelial growth factor (VEGF), regulating the ratio of matrix metalloproteinases (MMPs) and tissue inhibitor of metalloproteinases (TIMPs), as well as regulating the ratio of PR-A and PR-B expression within uterine fibroid cells and limiting its collagen overexpression [52,53].

Women receiving a 5 mg/d or 10 mg/d dosage notice a stop of menstrual bleeding within 1 week, varying from 81% to 90%, respectively [53]. A double-blind RCT published in 2015 showed a decrease of 54% and 58% in fibroid size when administrated to 5 mg/d and 10 mg/d doses of UPA, respectively, for 12 weeks [21]. Consequently, it seems the 5 mg/d and 10 mg/d doses both have similar efficacy [35]. The PEARL-II trial investigated matching UPA to the GnRH agonist leuprolide. The study determined that UPA was chosen owing to its strength to quickly decrease HMB (at 6 days versus 1 month) and the absence of hypoestrogenic signs [35]. Until now, the focus of medical treatment was usually short-term or preoperative therapy. However, developing data have recommended that UPA has the potential to be a long-term management choice, up to four cycles, 3 months each, for women with symptomatic uterine fibroids [58]. Of note, a study published in 2017 recommended that the absence of response to UPA in presumed fibroids should warrant a doubt for the presence of a malignant leiomyosarcoma [54].

The first U.S.-based phase III clinical trial (VENUS 1 study) was completed to evaluate the effectiveness and safety of UPA (5 and 10 mg) versus a placebo. The targets were amenorrhea and activity rate in premenopausal women. It showed promising findings regarding the rate of and time to amenorrhea without any adverse concerns that warranted discontinuation of the drug [55]. In the same study, the potency of UPA for fibroid treatment was investigated in different racial (Black versus non-Black) and body mass index (BMI) (30 kg/m^2 or greater versus less than 30 kg/m^2) groups with results highlighting the efficacy of UPA regardless of race and BMI [55].

Asoprisnil was first shown to repress uterine bleeding through a dual mechanism that includes a direct effect on the endometrium and inhibition of ovulation. However, it reduces bleeding at doses that did not inhibit ovulation, which means that the endometrial effects are the primary mechanism of bleeding suppression. The rapid effect on bleeding versus a gradual decrease in fibroid mass shows that the effect of PRMs on bleeding is independent of its effects on uterine fibroids [38,39]. Asoprisnil overcomes uterine bleeding in a dose-dependent way, and the reduced bleeding listed in 28%, 64%, and 83% of cases at 5, 10, and 25 mg/day, respectively, and diminished fibroid size by up to 36% at 25 mg/day, probably by minimizing uterine artery blood flow. Recently, follow-up studies have raised concerns about asoprisnil, because its primary function is as a progesterone antagonist, and it does not have an estrogenic effect in the endometrium [38]. Furthermore, clinical trials of telapristone acetate were suspended due to liver toxicity; however, trials have recently continued using lower doses of telapristone acetate [56]. At the molecular level, it works by the following mechanisms: inhibition of collagen synthesis that leads to apoptosis in uterine fibroids but does not affect normal myometrium [57]; reduction of the expression of antiapoptotic Bcl-2; increase in caspase-3; and attenuation of VEGF and proliferating cell nuclear antigen (PCNA) [58]. A multicenter, randomized placebo controlled trial found that after 12 weeks treatment with Asoprinil showed significant reduction in uterine bleeding, reduction in fibroid sizes with minimum hypoestrogenic side effect. Unluckily, recently due to the failing phase III clinical trial in 2008, it has not been taken more in clinical trials, due to unsafe changes in the endometrial lining of the uterus. Telapristone acetate (CDB4124), marked under the name of Proellex, has been tested as a treatment for symptoms linked to endometriosis and fibroid [59]. It showed encouraging findings in preliminary studies, successfully causing apoptosis in fibroid cells without affecting normal adjacent myometrium [59]. Researchers were expecting that telapristone could potentially become a long-term treatment. However, phase III studies were halted because of significant increases in liver enzymes [60]. Recently, there is a continuing phase II clinical trial that began in 2014 aiming to evaluate both safety and efficiency of lower oral as well as vaginal doses of telapristone acetate [64].

Vilaprisan (BAY 1002670) is a novel and highly effective SPRM with oral administration. Because of its pharmacological profile, this molecule is a promising drug in the regimen of many gynecological conditions. It is currently under evaluation for the long-term treatment of symptomatic fibroids [61]. In preclinical *in vitro* studies, vilaprisan showed strong selective binding activity to PR, exerting strong antagonism without agonistic activity. Vilaprisan can weakly bind glucocorticoid receptors (GRs), with a slight antiglucocorticoid effect (approximately 100 times less than mifepristone). Neither agonistic nor antagonistic activity has been observed on PR, and a very weak binding affinity has been detected for the androgen receptor (AR) [61,62]. Vilaprisan passed a 12-week phase I clinical trial successfully, in which most of the women who administrated the prescription daily at the dosage of 0.5–5 mg were able to reduce mean maximum serum concentrations of luteinizing hormone (LH) and follicle-stimulating hormone (FSH) and decrease mean and mean maximum estradiol concentrations [63]. Amenorrhea occurred in 75% of women at the doses of 1, 2, and 4 mg. These results confirmed the preliminaries of advanced clinical trials to evaluate vilaprisan in women with symptomatic fibroids [61,64]. In phase II, vilaprisan has been estimated at the doses of 0.5, 1, 2, and 4 mg daily for 12 weeks, in a double-blind, placebo-controlled study, and it was shown to manage bleeding within 3 days in most of the women at doses equal to or greater than 1 mg, and to obtain amenorrhea in 87%–92% of cases. Furthermore, improvements in symptoms related to fibroids and the quality of life were observed in all treatment groups and a dose-dependent volume reduction of fibroids up to 40% at the highest doses [65]. The same study shows that the reduction of bleeding and amenorrhea have been recoded within 3 days from the start of vilaprisan treatment [65]. The phase II study ASTEROID 2 (ClinicalTrials.gov Identifier: NCT02465814), for the first time, evaluated the efficacy and safety of different treatment regimens with vilaprisan at the daily doses of 2 mg (12 weeks of repeated cycles or 24 weeks of continuous treatment) compared to both placebo and UPA. The study was performed in patients with massive bleeding associated with uterine fibroids [60]. The study was completed at the end of 2016. Vilaprisan is currently under study in phase III for the long-term treatment of uterine fibroids, with the trials ASTEROID5 and ASTEROID6 (ClinicalTrials.

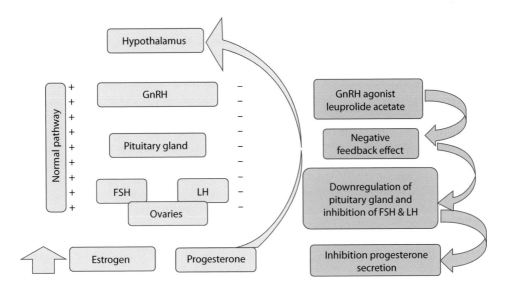

FIGURE 6.3 Treatment of uterine fibroids by gonadotropin-releasing hormone (GnRHa) agonist by initially increasing levels of follicle-stimulating hormone and luteinizing hormone, which elevate progesterone level and then subsequently suppress the release of GnRH through a negative feedback mechanism.

gov Identifier: NCT03240523 and NCT03194646, respectively). The study plan recommends evaluation of the efficiency and safety of vilaprisan 2 mg at different regimens, recruiting more than 3600 women worldwide; efficacy outcomes will be bleeding control, shrinkage in fibroid volume, and enhancement in the quality of life [61].

Gonadotropin-Releasing Hormone Agonist

Natural GnRH agonist was considered as one of the first therapeutic regimens to manage fibroids. GnRH stimulates gonadotrophs of the anterior pituitary and has been used for induction of ovulation. The GnRH agonists are highly potent and have an extended half-life compared to native GnRH. They produce an initial stimulation of pituitary gonadotrophs, which results in secretion of FSH and LH and the expected gonadal response. This response is accompanied by downregulation and inhibition of the pituitary-gonadal axis. As linked to GnRH agonists, GnRH antagonists immediately suppress pituitary gonadotropin by GnRH-receptor (GnRH-R) competition, through avoiding the initial stimulatory phase of the agonists [66] (Figure 6.3).

In 1999, leuprolide acetate (LA) was approved by the FDA as a short-term preoperative therapy to help women with symptomatic fibroid accompanied by anemia [67]. These compounds induce the hypoestrogenic effect by inhibition of the gonadal axis. The flare-up effect of GnRH by raise gonadotropin secretion, but after continuous secretions of GnRH leads to downregulation of GnRH receptors, consequently decrease, Stimulating follicle hormone (FSH) and luteinizing hormone (LH) thus putting the patients in pseudo-menopause state and reducing the size of fibroids and related symptoms. The main side effects of estrogen shortage are hot flashes, mood disturbance, and vaginal dryness, and the most serious effects are decreased BMD, which leads to restricting the use of LA, just for 3–6 months in the case used alone. Progestin-only, estrogen, progestin plus estrogen, and tibolone have been studied as add-back therapy. LA is considered expensive therapy compared with short-time treatment, and fibroids regrow to their original sizes after discontinuing the medication [68,69].

Developing New Medical Treatment for Uterine Fibroids

Nonpeptide Oral Gonadotropin-Releasing Hormone Antagonists

GnRH is a peptide that activates the pituitary to secrete hormones that are responsible for sex steroid reproduction and normal reproductive function. The search for nonpeptide, orally active GnRH antagonists has been launched by numerous pharmaceutical and biotechnology companies in the past two decades to overcome the problems associated with injectable GnRH antagonists and to perform a dose-dependent suppression of sex steroids [28,70]. Currently, three new nonpeptide GnRH antagonists, elagolix, relugolix, and OBE2109 (ObsEva), are for the control of fibroids and endometriosis [28]. These agents are short-acting, competitive antagonists of GnRH at the pituitary GnRH-R that reversibly inhibit receptor signaling, leading to dose-dependent suppression of LH and FSH, and, consequently, exhibit a dose-dependent suppression of ovarian and testicular sex steroids (Figure 6.4). The onset and discontinuance of these effects are rapid, in contrast to GnRH agonists' effects that induce hormonal suppression via desensitization of GnRH-R, as explained earlier. FDA has Oriahnn (elagolix with estradiol and norethindrone acetate) for the management of heavy menstrual bleeding associated with uterine fibroids on May 29, 2020. Oriahnn Elagolix is the first nonpeptide GnRH antagonist that has entered clinical development for hormone-dependent diseases in women. In phase I studies, treatment with elagolix showed a dose-dependent suppression of both gonadotropins and ovarian sex steroids in healthy premenopausal women [72]. A more recent phase I study, which incorporated a wide range of elagolix doses, indicated that elagolix could provide a dose-dependent estrogen inhibition, varying from partial suppression at a lower dose (150 mg once daily) to near-full suppression at higher doses (200– 300 mg twice daily) [72]. Estrogen suppression by high-dose elagolix is less than the estrogen suppression by depot GnRH agonists, which lower estradiol levels to post ovariectomy levels (less than 10 pg/mL). Elagolix has been evaluated in several randomized, controlled phase II studies in women with endometriosis and has shown a significant improvement in dysmenorrhea and nonmenstrual pelvic pain versus placebo in addition to an adequate safety and tolerability profile at a dose of 150 mg once daily [62]. Recently, the outcomes of randomized placebo-controlled phase III studies of 6 months' duration showed that elagolix (150 once daily and 200 mg twice daily) significantly and dose-dependently decreased dysmenorrhea, nonmenstrual pelvic pain, and dyspareunia versus placebo [73]. Harmonious with the mechanism of action, elagolix treatment was also associated with hypoestrogenic side effects (mainly hot flushes) and a decrease in BMD in a dose-dependent manner. Elagolix has been approved

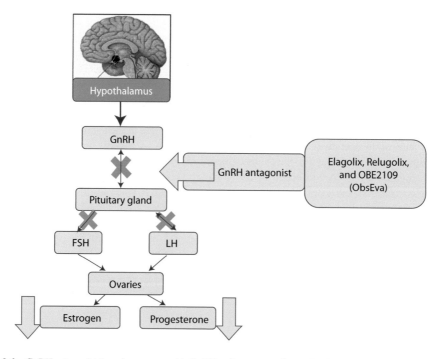

FIGURE 6.4 GnRH antagonist ligands compete with GnRH at the receptor site on the pituitary gonadotroph cell membrane leading to immediate suppression of the release of follicle-stimulating hormone and luteinizing hormone, which suppresses the release of progesterone.

for the management of HMB in women associated with uterine fibroids. The safety and efficacy of elagolix versus placebo and elagolix at various doses, with and without low-dose estradiol/progestogen add-back therapy, were estimated in a dose-finding, phase IIa study in women with HMB associated with uterine fibroids [74]. The objective alkaline hematin method was used for HMB assessment in this study, and a dose-dependent improvement in HMB with elagolix in women with fibroids was described. At month 3 of treatment with a 300-mg twice-daily dose, a 98% decline from baseline in MBL was shown. The low-dose add-back regimens (continuous/combined 1 mg estradiol/0.5 mg norethindrone acetate, and 1 mg estradiol acetate/200 mg cyclical progesterone) had minimal effects on HMB but mainly reduced the frequency of hot flushes. These results provided a reason for subsequent phase IIb and three clinical trials of longer duration as a potential long-term treatment of uterine fibroids in women experiencing HMB. This study also demonstrated, for the first time, the usefulness of low-dose estradiol (E2)/norethindrone acetate (NETA) add-back treatment in combination with a hormonally suppressive therapy in women with HMB and fibroids [73]. This placebo-controlled randomized study of 6 months' duration showed that elagolix, with or without two strengths of E2/NETA add-back therapy, significantly reduced MBL in uterine fibroid–associated HMB. Hot flushes and BMD were decreased by add-back therapy in a dose-dependent manner, but there is no statistically significant difference in BMD between elagolix plus the standard dose (1 mg E2/0.5 mg NETA as add-back group and the placebo group at month 6).

Relugolix

Relugolix is an orally active nonpeptide GnRH-receptor antagonist used for the treatment of different sex hormone–related dysfunctions. The medication inhibits the release of gonadotropin from the pituitary, leading to reductions of estradiol, progesterone, and testosterone levels, without producing the initial upregulation of hormone levels associated with GnRH agonists such as leuprorelin. Relugolix was later approved for marketing in Japan as a medication for symptoms associated with uterine fibroids, and studies estimating the efficacy of the agent as a treatment for endometriosis-associated pain and prostate cancer have begun. The approved adult dosage of relugolix in Japan is 40 mg once daily, orally administered [76,77].

Statins

There is evidence that the antihyperlipidemic drug simvastatin and other drugs from the same family may represent a medical treatment option for uterine fibroids [78,79]. Borahay et al. showed that it inhibits proliferation of fibroid cells and induces apoptosis through calcium-dependent mechanisms [80]. In addition, the same group also demonstrated that it inhibits fibroid tumor growth in a patient-derived xenograft animal model [81]. Another group demonstrated that another similar drug, atorvastatin, suppresses uterine fibroid tumor growth [82]. Using epidemiologic (insurance claims) data, statins were noted to be associated with a lower incidence of uterine fibroids and fibroid-associated symptoms and myomectomies [83]. Malik et al. also showed that simvastatin at low doses can inhibit production of extracellular matrix proteins in uterine fibroids [75]. There is currently an ongoing clinical trial for simvastatin in patients with uterine fibroids.

Conclusions and Future Directions

Currently, available treatment options are restricted, and approved market medications are often used for short-term treatment to control HMB. Progestogens and COCs usually provide a brief improvement in HMB. The LNG-IUS is valuable in decreasing bleeding, but it is used only in women with a normal uterine cavity. These medications reduce bleeding by targeting the endometrium and do not diminish fibroid volume. GnRH agonists are highly effective in suppressing bleeding and reducing fibroids and uterine mass. Leuprolide acetate is FDA approved for presurgery short-term treatment. No hormonal add-back therapies have been approved as GnRH agonists for long-term treatment of fibroids. However, some medications currently under investigation in the United States, such as PRMs and oral GnRH antagonists, offer a promise of new fertility-sparing medical therapies that could provide a long-term treatment option for women with fibroids. Alternative treatment using UPA has recently been approved in Europe and Canada for the long-term management of symptomatic fibroids. Vilaprisan has been evaluated only in women with symptomatic fibroids, and it has an advantage over other SPRMs, such as UPA. Vilaprisan exhibits more rapid action on bleeding related to fibroids but shows effects with lower doses than other SPRMs. Elagolix is an FDA-approved oral treatment for controlling endometriosis with symptoms from a moderate to severe degree. A recent phase IIb study of therapy with elagolix combined with low-dose add-back therapy exhibited high efficiency and improvements in HMB. This combination treatment shows a low rate of hypoestrogenic side effects such as vasomotor signs and changes in BMD. Continuous studies of the pathogenesis of uterine fibroids and a new pharmacological target, nonhormonal effect, and long-term medical regimen to eradicate this disease are needed.

Conflict of Interest

Ayman Al-Hendy is a consultant for Allergan plc, Bayer, Repros, and AbbVie.

REFERENCES

1. Al-Hendy A and Salama S. Gene therapy and uterine leiomyoma: A review. *Hum Reprod Update.* 2006;12(4):385–400.
2. Elkafas H, Qiwei Y, and Al-Hendy A. Origin of uterine fibroids: Conversion of myometrial stem cells to tumor-initiating cells. *Semin Reprod Med.* 2017;35(6):481–6.
3. Yang Q, Mas A, Diamond MP, and Al-Hendy A. The mechanism and function of epigenetics in uterine leiomyoma development. *Reprod Sci.* 2016;23(2):163–75.
4. Mas A, Stone L, O'Connor PM et al. Developmental exposure to endocrine disruptors expands murine myometrial stem cell compartment as a prerequisite to leiomyoma tumorigenesis. *Stem Cells.* 2017;35(3):666–78.
5. Wilson AC, Meethal SV, Bowen RL, and Atwood CS. Leuprolide acetate: A drug of diverse clinical applications. *Expert Opin Investig Drugs.* 2007;16(11):1851–63.
6. Ishikawa H, Ishi K, Serna VA, Kakazu R, Bulun SE, and Kurita T. Progesterone is essential for maintenance and growth of uterine leiomyoma. *Endocrinology.* 2010;151(6):2433–42.
7. Markowski DN, von Ahsen I, Nezhad MH, Wosniok W, Helmke BM, and Bullerdiek J. HMGA2 and the p19Arf-TP53-CDKN1A axis: A delicate balance in the growth of uterine leiomyomas. *Genes Chromosomes Cancer.* 2010;49(8):661–8.
8. Makinen N, Mehine M, Tolvanen J et al. MED12, the mediator complex subunit 12 gene, is mutated at high frequency in uterine leiomyomas. *Science.* 2011;334(6053):252–5.
9. Markowski DN, Bartnitzke S, Löning T, Drieschner N, Helmke BM, and Bullerdiek J. MED12 mutations in uterine fibroids—their relationship to cytogenetic subgroups. *International Journal of Cancer.* 2012; 131(7):1528–36.
10. Medikare V, Kandukuri LR, Ananthapur V, Deenadayal M, and Nallari P. The genetic bases of uterine fibroids; a review. *Journal of Reproduction & Infertility.* 2011;12(13):1.
11. Elkafas H, Ali M, Elmorsy E, Kamel R, Thompson WE, Badary O. Al-Hendy A, and Yang Q. Vitamin D3 ameliorates DNA damage caused by developmental exposure to endocrine disruptors in the uterine myometrial stem cells of Eker rats. *Cells.* 2020;9(6):1469.
12. Prusinski Fernung LE, Yang Q, Sakamuro D, Kumari A, Mas A, and Al-Hendy A. Endocrine disruptor exposure during development increases incidence of uterine fibroids by altering DNA repair in myometrial stem cells. *Biology of Reproduction.* 2018;99(4):735–48.
13. Prusinski L, Al-Hendy A, and Yang Q. Developmental exposure to endocrine disrupting chemicals alters the epigenome: Identification of reprogrammed targets. *Gynecol Obstet Res Open J.* 2016;3(1):1–6.
14. Pavone D, Clemenza S, Sorbi F, Fambrini M, and Petraglia F. Epidemiology and risk factors of uterine fibroids. *Best Pract Res Clin Obstet Gynaecol.* 2018;46:3–11.
15. Parazzini F. Risk factors for clinically diagnosed uterine fibroids in women around menopause. *Maturitas.* 2006;55(2):174–9.

16. Baird DD, Kesner JS, and Dunson DB. Luteinizing hormone in premenopausal women may stimulate uterine leiomyomata development. *J Soc Gynecol Investig.* 2006;13(2):130–5.

17. Al-Hendy A, Diamond MP, El-Sohemy A, and Halder SK. 1,25–dihydroxyvitamin D3 regulates expression of sex steroid receptors in human uterine fibroid cells. *J Clin Endocrinol Metab.* 2015;100(4): E572–82.

18. Moravek MB, Yin P, Ono M et al. Ovarian steroids, stem cells and uterine leiomyoma: Therapeutic implications. *Hum Reprod Update.* 2015;21(1):1–12.

19. Katz TA, Yang Q, Treviño LS, Walker CL, and Al-Hendy A. Endocrine-disrupting chemicals and uterine fibroids. *Fertil Steril.* 2016;106(4):967–77.

20. Stewart L, Glenn GM, Stratton P et al. Association of germline mutations in the fumarate hydratase gene and uterine fibroids in women with hereditary leiomyomatosis and renal cell cancer. *Arch Dermatol.* 2008;144(12):1584–92.

21. Patel B, Elguero S, Thakore S, Dahoud W, Bedaiwy M, and Mesiano S. Role of nuclear progesterone receptor isoforms in uterine pathophysiology. *Hum Reprod Update.* 2015;21(2):155–73.

22. Al-Hendy A, Diamond MP, Boyer TG, and Halder SK. Vitamin D3 inhibits Wnt/beta-catenin and mTOR signaling pathways in human uterine fibroid cells. *J Clin Endocrinol Metab.* 2016;101(4):1542–51.

23. Goyeneche AA and Telleria CM. Antiprogestins in gynecological diseases. *Reproduction.* 2015;149(1):R15–33.

24. Clarke-Pearson DL and Geller EJ. Complications of hysterectomy. *Obstet Gynecol.* 2013;121(3):654–73.

25. Donnez J, Donnez O, Courtoy GE, and Dolmans M-M. The place of selective progesterone receptor modulators in myoma therapy. *Minerva Ginecol.* 2016;68(3):313–20.

26. Donnez J and Dolmans M-M. Uterine fibroid management: From the present to the future. *Hum Reprod Update.* 2016;22(6):665–86.

27. Ali M, Chaudhry ZT, and Al-Hendy A. Successes and failures of uterine leiomyoma drug discovery. *Expert Opin Drug Discov.* 2018;13(2):169–77.

28. Chwalisz K and Taylor H. Current and emerging medical treatments for uterine fibroids. *Semin Reprod Med.* 2017;35(6):510–22.

29. National Collaborating Centre for Women's and Children's Health. *National Institute for Health and Clinical Excellence: Guidance. Heavy Menstrual Bleeding.* London: RCOG Press National Collaborating Centre for Women's and Children's Health; 2007.

30. Irvine GA, Campbell-Brown MB, Lumsden MA, Heikkila A, Walker JJ, and Cameron IT. Randomised comparative trial of the levonorgestrel intrauterine system and norethisterone for treatment of idiopathic menorrhagia. *Br J Obstet Gynaecol.* 1998;105(6):592–8.

31. Sangkomkamhang US, Lumbiganon P, Laopaiboon M, and Mol BW. Progestogens or progestogen-releasing intrauterine systems for uterine fibroids. *Cochrane Database Syst Rev.* 2013;(2):CD008994.

32. Carr BR, Marshburn PB, Weatherall PT et al. An evaluation of the effect of gonadotropin-releasing hormone analogs and medroxyprogesterone acetate on uterine leiomyomata volume by magnetic resonance imaging: A prospective, randomized, double blind, placebo-controlled, crossover trial. *J Clin Endocrinol Metab.* 1993;76(5):1217–23.

33. Rogers P, Martinez F, Girling J et al. Influence of different hormonal regimens on endometrial microvascular density and VEGF expression in women suffering from breakthrough bleeding. *Hum Reprod.* 2005;20(12):3341–7.

34. Spitz IM (ed). *Progesterone Receptor Antagonists and Selective Progesterone Receptor Modulators (SPRMs). Seminars in Reproductive Medicine.* New York, NY: Thieme Medical Publishers; 2005.

35. Chabbert-Buffet N, Meduri G, Bouchard P, and Spitz IM. Selective progesterone receptor modulators and progesterone antagonists: Mechanisms of action and clinical applications. *Hum Reprod Update.* 2005;11(3):293–307.

36. Chwalisz K, Perez MC, Demanno D, Winkel C, Schubert G, and Elger W. Selective progesterone receptor modulator development and use in the treatment of leiomyomata and endometriosis. *Endocr Rev.* 2005;26(3):423–38.

37. Elger W, Fähnrich M, Beier S, Qing SS, and Chwalisz K. Endometrial and myometrial effects of progesterone antagonists in pregnant guinea pigs. *J Obstet Gynaecol.* 1987;157(4):1065–74.

38. Chwalisz K, Larsen L, Mattia-Goldberg C, Edmonds A, Elger W, and Winkel CA. A randomized, controlled trial of asoprisnil, a novel selective progesterone receptor modulator, in women with uterine leiomyomata. *Fertil Steril.* 2007;87(6):1399–412.

39. Donnez J, Tatarchuk TF, Bouchard P et al. Ulipristal acetate versus placebo for fibroid treatment before surgery. *N Engl J Med.* 2012;366(5):409–20.

40. Bartels CB, Cayton KC, Chuong FS et al. An evidence-based approach to the medical management of fibroids: A systematic review. *Clin Obstet Gynecol.* 2016;59(1):30–52.

41. Murji A, Whitaker L, Chow TL, and Sobel ML. Selective progesterone receptor modulators (SPRMs) for uterine fibroids. *Cochrane Database Syst Rev.* 2017;Issue 4. Art. No. CD010770.

42. Faustino F, Martinho M, Reis J, and Águas F. Update on medical treatment of uterine fibroids. *Eur J Obstet Gynecol Reprod Biol.* 2017;216:61–8.

43. Talaulikar VS and Manyonda I. Progesterone and progesterone receptor modulators in the management of symptomatic uterine fibroids. *Eur J Obstet Gynecol Reprod Biol.* 2012;165(2):135–40.

44. Eisinger SH, Fiscella J, Bonfiglio T, Meldrum S, and Fiscella K. Open-label study of ultra low-dose mifepristone for the treatment of uterine leiomyomata. *Eur J Obstet Gynecol Reprod Biol.* 2009;146(2):215–8.

45. Islam MS, Protic O, Giannubilo SR et al. Uterine leiomyoma: Available medical treatments and new possible therapeutic options. *J Clin Endocrinol Metab.* 2013;98(3):921–34.

46. Shen Q, Hua Y, Jiang W, Zhang W, Chen M, and Zhu X. Effects of mifepristone on uterine leiomyoma in premenopausal women: A meta-analysis. *Fertil Steril.* 2013;100(6):1722–6.e10.

47. Ciarmela P, Islam MS, Reis FM et al. Growth factors and myometrium: Biological effects in uterine fibroid and possible clinical implications. *Hum Reprod Update.* 2011;17(6):772–90.

48. Freed MM and Spies JB (eds). *Uterine Artery Embolization for Fibroids: A Review of Current Outcomes. Seminars in Reproductive Medicine.* New York, NY: Thieme Medical Publishers; 2010.

49. Torre A, Paillusson B, Fain V, Labauge P, Pelage J, and Fauconnier A. Uterine artery embolization for severe symptomatic fibroids: Effects on fertility and symptoms. *Hum Reprod.* 2014;29(3):490–501.

50. Talaulikar VS and Manyonda IT. Ulipristal acetate: A novel option for the medical management of symptomatic uterine fibroids. *Adv Ther.* 2012;29(8):655–63.

51. Ohara N, Morikawa A, Chen W et al. Comparative effects of SPRM asoprisnil (J867) on proliferation, apoptosis, and the expression of growth factors in cultured uterine leiomyoma cells and normal myometrial cells. *Reprod Sci.* 2007;14(suppl 8):20–7.

52. Fujimoto J, Hirose R, Ichigo S, Sakaguchi H, Li Y, and Tamaya T. Expression of progesterone receptor form A and B mRNAs in uterine leiomyoma. *Tumor Biol.* 1998;19(2):126–31.

53. Maruo T, Ohara N, Yoshida S et al. Lessons learned from the preclinical drug discovery of asoprisnil and ulipristal for non-surgical treatment of uterine leiomyomas. *Expert Opin Drug Discov.* 2011;6(9):897–911.

54. Kadhel P, Smail M, and De Mozota DB. Inefficiency of ulipristal acetate on uterus leiomyomas as an additional sign to suspect leiomyosarcoma. *J Gynecol Obstet Hum Reprod.* 2017;46(7):609–11.

55. Simon J, Catherino W, Segars J et al. First US-based phase 3 study of ulipristal acetate (UPA) for symptomatic uterine fibroids (UF): Results of VENUS-I. *Fertil Steril.* 2016;106(3):e376.

56. Bouchard P, Chabbert-Buffet N, and Fauser BC. Selective progesterone receptor modulators in reproductive medicine: Pharmacology, clinical efficacy and safety. *Fertil Steril.* 2011;96(5):1175–89.

57. Donnez J, Donnez O, and Dolmans MM. With the advent of selective progesterone receptor modulators, what is the place of myoma surgery in current practice? *Fertil Steril.* 2014;102(3):640–8.

58. Kashani BN, Centini G, Morelli SS, Weiss G, and Petraglia F. Role of medical management for uterine leiomyomas. *Best Pract Res Clin Obstet Gynaecol.* 2016;34:85–103.

59. Luo X, Yin P, Coon VJ, Cheng YH, Wiehle RD, and Bulun SE. The selective progesterone receptor modulator CDB4124 inhibits proliferation and induces apoptosis in uterine leiomyoma cells. *Fertil Steril.* 2010;93(8):2668–73.

60. Goenka L, George M, and Sen M. A peek into the drug development scenario of endometriosis—A systematic review. *Biomed Pharmacother.* 2017;90:575–85.

61. Melis GB, Neri M, Piras B et al. Vilaprisan for treating uterine fibroids. *Expert Opin Investig Drugs.* 2018;27(5):497–505.

62. Diamond MP, Carr B, Dmowski WP et al. Elagolix treatment for endometriosis-associated pain: Results from a phase 2, randomized, double-blind, placebo-controlled study. *Reprod Sci.* 2014;21(3):363–71.

63. Schutt B, Kaiser A, Schultze-Mosgau MH et al. Pharmacodynamics and safety of the novel selective progesterone receptor modulator vilaprisan: A double-blind, randomized, placebo-controlled phase 1 trial in healthy women. *Hum Reprod.* 2016;31(8):1703–12.

64. Bouchard P and Chabbert-Buffet N. The history and use of the progesterone receptor modulator ulipristal acetate for heavy menstrual bleeding with uterine fibroids. *Best Pract Res Clin Obstet Gynaecol.* 2017;40:105–10.

65. Seitz C, Bumbuliene Z, Costa AR et al. Rationale and design of ASTEROID 2, a randomized, placebo- and active comparator-controlled study to assess the efficacy and safety of vilaprisan in patients with uterine fibroids. *Contemp Clin Trials.* 2017;55:56–62.

66. Kumar P and Sharma A. Gonadotropin-releasing hormone analogs: Understanding advantages and limitations. *J Hum Reprod Sci.* 2014;7(3):170.

67. Segars JH, Parrott EC, Nagel JD et al. Proceedings from the Third National Institutes of Health International Congress on Advances in Uterine Leiomyoma Research: Comprehensive review, conference summary and future recommendations. *Hum Reprod Update.* 2014;20(3):309–33.

68. Morris EP, Rymer J, Robinson J, and Fogelman I. Efficacy of tibolone as "add-back therapy" in conjunction with a gonadotropin-releasing hormone analogue in the treatment of uterine fibroids. *Fertil Steril.* 2008;89(2):421–8.

69. Moroni RM, Martins WP, Ferriani RA et al. Add-back therapy with GnRH analogues for uterine fibroids. *Cochrane Database Syst Rev.* 2015(3):CD010854.

70. Millar RP and Newton CL. Current and future applications of GnRH, kisspeptin and neurokinin B analogues. *Nat Rev Endocrinol.* 2013;9(8):451–66.

71. Choy M. Pharmaceutical approval update. *P & T: A Peer-Reviewed Journal for Formulary Management.* 2018;43(10):599–628.

72. Ng J, Chwalisz K, Carter DC, and Klein CE. Dose-dependent suppression of gonadotropins and ovarian hormones by elagolix in healthy premenopausal women. *J Clin Endocrinol Metab.* 2017;102(5):1683–91.

73. Taylor HS, Giudice LC, Lessey BA et al. Treatment of endometriosis-associated pain with Elagolix, an oral GnRH antagonist. *N Engl J Med.* 2017;377(1):28–40.

74. Archer DF, Stewart EA, Jain RI et al. Elagolix for the management of heavy menstrual bleeding associated with uterine fibroids: Results from a phase 2a proof-of-concept study. *Fertil Steril.* 2017;108(1):152–60.e4.

75. Malik M, Britten J, Borahay M, Segars J, and Catherino WH. Simvastatin, at clinically relevant concentrations, affects human uterine leiomyoma growth and extracellular matrix production. *Fertil Steril.* 2018;110(7):1398–407e1.

76. Markham A. Relugolix: First global approval. *Drugs.* 2019;79(6):675–9.

77. MacLean DB, Shi H, Faessel HM, and Saad F. Medical castration using the investigational oral GnRH antagonist TAK-385 (Relugolix): Phase 1 study in healthy males. *J Clin Endocrinol Metab.* 2015;100(12):4579–87.

78. Fritton K and Borahay MA. New and emerging therapies for uterine fibroids. *Semin Reprod Med.* 2017;35(6):549–59.

79. Zeybek B, Costantine M, Kilic GS, and Borahay MA. Therapeutic roles of statins in gynecology and obstetrics: The current evidence. *Reprod Sci.* 2018;25(6):802–17.

80. Borahay MA, Kilic GS, Yallampalli C et al. Simvastatin potently induces calcium-dependent apoptosis of human leiomyoma cells. *J Biol Chem.* 2014;289(51):35075–86.

81. Borahay MA, Vincent K, Motamedi M et al. Novel effects of simvastatin on uterine fibroids: In vitro and patient-derived xenograft mouse model study. *Am J Obstet Gynecol.* 2015;213(2):196.e1–e8.

82. Shen Z, Li S, Sheng B et al. The role of atorvastatin in suppressing tumor growth of uterine fibroids. *J Transl Med.* 2018;16(1):53.

83. Borahay MA, Fang X, Baillargeon JG, Kilic GS, Boehning DF, and Kuo YF. Statin use and uterine fibroid risk in hyperlipidemia patients: A nested case-control study. *Am J Obstet Gynecol.* 2016;215(6):750.e1–e8.

84. Elhusseini H, Elkafas H, Abdelaziz M et al. Diet-induced vitamin D deficiency triggers inflammation and DNA damage profile in murine myometrium. *International Journal of Women's Health.* 2018;10:503–14.

7

Fibroid Preoperative Imaging: Ultrasound

Nicole Catherine Michel, Shima Albasha, and Botros R.M.B. Rizk

CONTENTS

Introduction

Fibroids are the most prevalent type of benign tumors of the uterus among reproductive-aged women. They arise primarily from smooth muscle cells of the myometrium and affect almost one-third of women over the age of 35 years [1–3]. Factors associated with a higher risk of developing fibroids include age, obesity, early menarche, nulliparity, race, genetic factors, and long-term hormonal therapy [4,5]. Although fibroids are asymptomatic in the majority of patients, they may cause menorrhagia, pelvic pressure, lumbar pain, urinary and bowel dysfunction, dyspareunia, and obstetric complications [6]. Three types of fibroids exist, and they are labeled according to their position in the uterine wall: submucosal, intramural, and subserosal [7]. Fibroid size, quantity, and location relative to the uterus are all valuable considerations. In the pregnant patient, the fibroid location relative to the placenta has even further significance, as it may possibly direct the course of action that the obstetrician decides to take [8].

Various imaging modalities can be utilized to assess the magnitude and position of tumors. Principally, two-dimensional (2D) ultrasonography (US) has provided an inexpensive, noninvasive means for diagnosing uterine fibroids for the past few decades. Thus, it is customarily the imaging modality that is used initially. More recently, the addition of three-dimensional (3D) ultrasound, color Doppler, and saline infusion sonohysterography (SIS) have enhanced the diagnostic capacity of US. SIS has been conducive to identifying localized intracavitary lesions [2]. This segment primarily examines use of US in preoperative imaging of uterine fibroids. Of note, the production of this section has greatly benefited from the work of Drs. Clough, Khalaf, Allahbadia, Merchant, Abuzeid, and Joseph [1–3].

Ultrasound Technique

Two-Dimensional Ultrasound

The traditional way to image fibroids is by 2D scanning. For good visualization of fibroids, specifically of the outline, the best imaging mode is the transvaginal scan (TVS). By this method, the probe is in closer proximity to the uterus, and a higher frequency can be selected, thereby yielding finer tissue delineation [1]. The rationale behind this can be elucidated by basic physics. Strictly speaking, ultrasounds adhere to the following general pattern: lower frequencies deliver sharpened resolution but are restricted in depth of penetration; the same can be expected vice versa [9]. Notably, an ultrasound is optimally executed if the patient has an empty bladder. TVS is conducted using a curved linear array endocavity transducer with a frequency range of 6–9 MHz [10]. Since fibroids are composed of mixed, dense tissue, they can be highly attenuating on ultrasound, resulting in obscurity and poor transmission. Therefore, it is necessary, at times, to choose a lower frequency to accommodate for better penetration, in order to observe the posterior aspect of a fibroid [6]. If a uterus is considerably enlarged by fibroids, to a point where TVS fails to expose the complete uterus, then a transabdominal scan (TAS) is needed. TAS is carried out using a curved linear array abdominal transducer that has an average frequency ranging from 2.5 to 5 MHz [11]. Along with modifying the frequency of the ultrasound, altering the harmonics and amplifying the power settings can also enhance the picture [12].

Two-dimensional ultrasound has even proven useful for tackling complex cases, such as those involving fibroids located on the broad ligament [3,13]. In one instance, Abuzeid and Joseph describe the case of a 31-year-old female with this condition who was being evaluated for infertility [3]. TVS revealed a right-sided broad ligament fibroid so immense that it drove the entire uterus toward the left side and inhabited most of the pelvic cavity (Figure 7.1a–c). The diagnosis was also confirmed on SIS with and without Doppler flow analysis (Figure 7.2a,b). It showed an expansion in the vascularity amidst the uterus and fibroid. The diagnosis was then substantiated via diagnostic laparoscopy (Figure 7.3). Following successful removal of the fibroid, this patient was able to conceive and give birth to a healthy child. This case is an excellent demonstration of the application of TVS in ascertaining the degree of attachment and vascularity of a broad ligament lesion. Such information is helpful in guiding treatment planning [3].

Two-dimensional scanning is a conservative, noninvasive approach for the discovery of endometrial pathology in women with dysfunctional uterine bleeding. TVS is capable of rendering sufficient information to refrain from having an unnecessary hysteroscopy. Characteristically, in women who are postmenopausal, the endometrial thickness reliably identifies those who need further testing. Among this approximate age group, a thin endometrium is ordinarily promising and rules out pathology in the uterine cavity, namely, cancer [14].

Three-Dimensional Ultrasound

While 2D ultrasound is limited to representing a fibroid in the longitudinal and transverse planes, 3D scanning is able to display the fibroid in the coronal plane. This is exceptionally convenient when surveying a fibroid that is within, or impinging on, the cavity. Since the introduction of 3D technology, the 3D ultrasound has proven itself to be a useful tool for the exploration of uterine pathology, due to its power to reconstruct the coronal plane of the uterus [15]. Three-dimensional ultrasound has proven its efficiency in visualizing fibroids on a uterus with anatomical anomalies, such as in the case of an arcuate uterus or a uterine septum [3]. If there is solid image contrast between the fibroid and endometrial lining, then clear observation of the fibroid is more likely to be attained. Ideal contrast is presumed to be attained throughout the secretory phase of the cycle, when the endometrium appears hyperechoic (Figure 7.4).

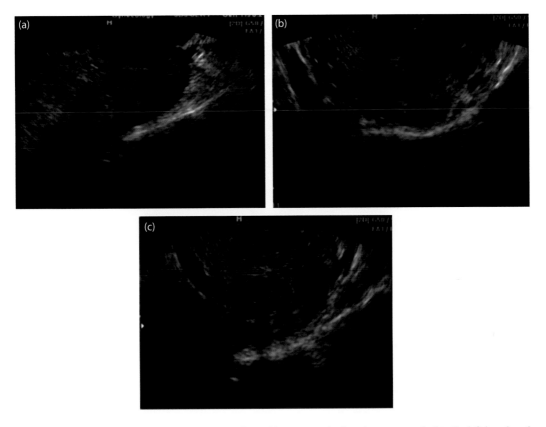

FIGURE 7.1 Transvaginal scan images demonstrating a (a) transverse look at the uterus pushed to the left by a broad ligament fibroid; (b) transverse view of a large uterine fibroid that inhabits almost the entire pelvic cavity; (c) transverse view of a large uterine fibroid with a sizable blood vessel fixed between the fibroid and pelvic sidewall. (From Abuzeid MI and Joseph SK. Trans-vaginal ultrasound scan findings: Effect on treatment plan. In: Rizk B and Puscheck E [eds] *Ultrasonography in Gynecology.* Cambridge, UK: Cambridge University Press; 2015, pp. 80–93. With permission.)

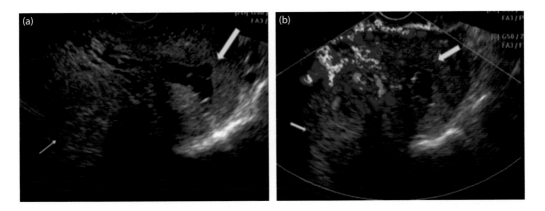

FIGURE 7.2 Saline infusion sonohysterography demonstrating a (a) transverse view of the uterus with normal endometrial cavity (large arrow) and a large broad ligament fibroid (small arrow); and (b) transverse view of the uterus with Doppler flow study showing a normal endometrial cavity (large arrow) and a large broad ligament fibroid (small arrow). In both images, note the considerable increase in vascularity between the uterus and fibroid. (From Abuzeid MI and Joseph SK. Trans-vaginal ultrasound scan findings: Effect on treatment plan. In: Rizk B and Puscheck E [eds] *Ultrasonography in Gynecology.* Cambridge, UK: Cambridge University Press; 2015, pp. 80–93. With permission.)

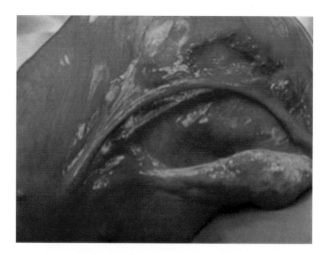

FIGURE 7.3 Laparoscopic image displaying a large broad ligament fibroid pushing the uterus to the left. Note that the right fallopian tube is extended and pulled over the fibroid. (From Abuzeid MI and Joseph SK. Trans-vaginal ultrasound scan findings: Effect on treatment plan. In: Rizk B, and Puscheck E [eds] *Ultrasonography in Gynecology.* Cambridge, UK: Cambridge University Press; 2015, pp. 80–93. With permission.)

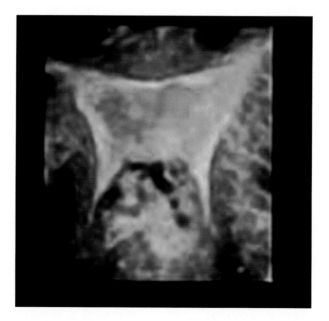

FIGURE 7.4 Three-dimensional coronal view of the uterus displaying a massive submucosal fibroid situated in the central region of the uterine cavity. (From Clough A and Khalaf Y. Ultrasonography of uterine fibroids. In: Rizk B [ed] *Ultrasonography in Reproductive Medicine and Infertility.* Cambridge, UK: Cambridge University Press; 2010, pp. 88–96. With permission.)

Saline Infusion Sonohysterography

Saline infusion sonohysterography (SIS) should be considered if US is not sufficiently helpful, or in the case of medical treatment failure. SIS has become a fundamental instrument, particularly in the assessment of cavity distortion caused by fibroids. This method involves injecting a small amount of saline into the uterine cavity via a uterine cannula. Following introduction of saline into the uterine cavity, US can delineate submucous myomas and indicate the proximity of intramural myomas to the endometrial cavity [15]. Studies have shown SIS to be useful in preoperative assessment, given that SIS can provide further information on size and location of submucosal fibroids in comparison with conventional US [16]. This is especially important, seeing as an exemplary preoperative assessment leads to a more accurate resection of fibroids. If a fibroid impinges on the cavity, then assessment is made of what percentage of the lesion projects into the cavity, and its degree of infiltration into the myometrium. Submucosal fibroids can then be categorized as type 0, 1, or 2 in terms of their extent of cavity distortion according to the classification system of the International Federation of Gynecology and Obstetrics (FIGO) [17]. Three-dimensional scanning can be performed together with SIS to provide the additional coronal plane for further diagnostic accuracy.

Hysterosalpingo Contrast Sonography

Hysterosalpingo contrast sonography (HyCoSy) is a well-tolerated procedure that is considered a first-line choice for evaluating tubal patency and for exploration of the uterine cavity in infertile women [18]. If a fibroid is located adjacent to the ostia, a HyCoSy test may help to determine whether the fibroid is causing an ostial obstruction, as indicated by a lack of cornual exit of contrast. Echovist (the contrast used for HyCoSy) also provides a "positive" contrast for precise demarcation of submucosal fibroids (Figure 7.5a–d).

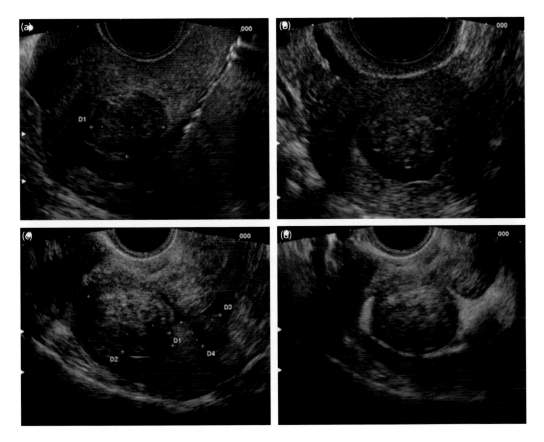

FIGURE 7.5 Saline infusion sonohysterography examinations of submucosal fibroids showing (a) type 2, (b) type 1, (c) type 0, and (d) type 0. (From Clough A and Khalaf Y. Ultrasonography of uterine fibroids. In: Rizk B [ed] *Ultrasonography in Reproductive Medicine and Infertility.* Cambridge, UK: Cambridge University Press; 2010, pp. 88–96. With permission.)

Color Doppler

Color Doppler can be beneficial in the evaluation of the fibroid blood supply. It is particularly helpful for spotting the pedicle attaching a fibroid to the uterus when there is doubt about the etiology of a fibroid lying within the pelvis. It can also be used to differentiate between an endometrial polyp and submucosal fibroid. The polyp vessels often have a central feeder vessel that diverges into smaller vessels. On the other hand, the blood vessels supplying the fibroid can be seen at its periphery [19]. Color Doppler is also useful for directing treatment plans, as well as for post-treatment follow-up for radiological treatment of fibroids, such as uterine artery embolization (UAE). Color Doppler is also exceptional at discerning fibroids from adenomyosis, which may be commonly mistaken [20]. Overall, when utilized in conjunction with color Doppler, TVS is the mainstay of initial management in the case of abnormal uterine bleeding, as it can dependably rule out the most common uterine pathologies, such as polyps and fibroids.

Magnetic Resonance Imaging

Magnetic resonance imaging (MRI) is an esteemed alternative imaging modality that offers decent soft tissue contrast and is more sensitive to uncovering pathology than US [21]. A noteworthy capability of MRI is its accuracy in mapping fibroids for preoperatively planning for treatment of symptomatic fibroids via UAE [22]. However, the higher cost and lower availability of MRI can be a setback. Hence, MRI is generally only used for complex cases.

Establishing a Correct Diagnosis via Ultrasound

Ultrasound Features of Fibroids

Fibroids can be appreciated on ultrasound as having a round silhouette and heterogeneity (Figure 7.6a–d). They normally present as distinct, hypoechoic lesions that generate a variable extent of acoustic shadowing on ultrasound [23]. Fibroids may make the uterus look immense or may distort the natural uterine contour. Even though noncalcified fibroids frequently demonstrate some posterior acoustic shadowing, this is certainly more pronounced in fibroids that are calcified [24].

For reference, intraoperative photos of gross fibroid lesions can be seen in Figure 7.7.

With regard to treatment options for large fibroids, modern techniques that are commonly performed can be seen in Figures 7.8a–d and 7.9a–c.

Ultrasound Features of Various Differential Diagnoses

Adenomyosis

Adenomyosis is a benign condition in which endometrial cells are pathologically manifested in the myometrium of the uterus [25]. Like fibroids, adenomyosis is a prevalent diagnosis among women and raises similar symptoms of abnormal uterine bleeding and menstrual cramping. The initial imaging modality, TAS, might show enlargement of the uterus, or irregular thickening of the walls in the myometrium. US features of adenomyosis often consist of the following sonographic details: heterogenous reflectivity, changes in echogenicity, and myometrial cysts (Figure 7.10a). As opposed to fibroids, an adenomyoma is more elliptical shaped, with poorly demarcated edges, no calcifications, and no peripheral shadowing. In uncertain instances, Doppler sonography is often valuable. In an adenomyoma, blood vessels generally keep on their usual vertical course in the myometrial regions, while in the case of uterine fibroid, blood vessels are usually located in the periphery [26]. Of note, various studies have shown that adenomyosis regularly coexists with other gynecological conditions, like endometriosis and fibroids [27].

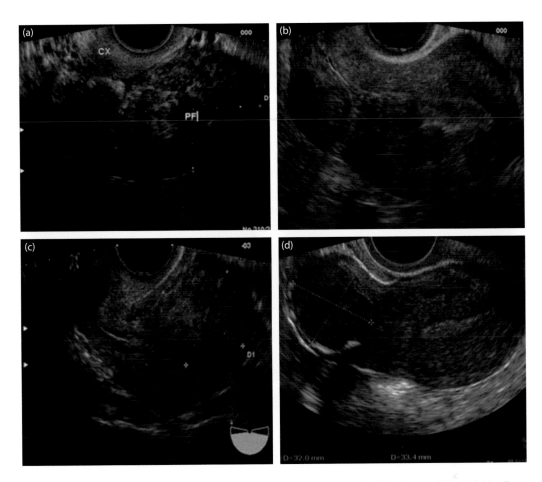

FIGURE 7.6 Ultrasound images of (a) pedunculated fibroid arising from the cervix; (b) submucosal fibroid (with adjacent intramural fibroid in the cervix); (c) intramural fibroid (with indeterminate intrusion on the cavity); and (d) subserosal fibroid. (From Clough A and Khalaf Y. Ultrasonography of uterine fibroids. In: Rizk B [ed] *Ultrasonography in Reproductive Medicine and Infertility.* Cambridge, UK: Cambridge University Press; 2010, pp. 88–96. With permission.)

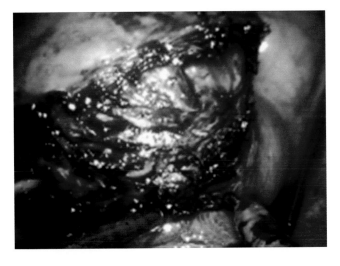

FIGURE 7.7 Large fibroid lesion. (Courtesy of Professor Botros Rizk.)

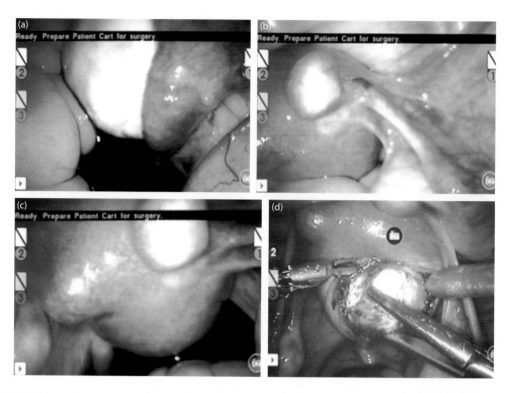

FIGURE 7.8 (a–d) Robotic myomectomy procedure for removal of fibroids. (Courtesy of Professor Botros Rizk.)

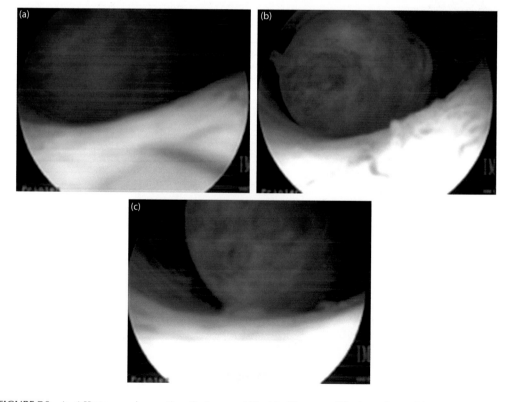

FIGURE 7.9 (a–c) Hysteroscopic resection of submucosal fibroids. (Courtesy of Professor Botros Rizk.)

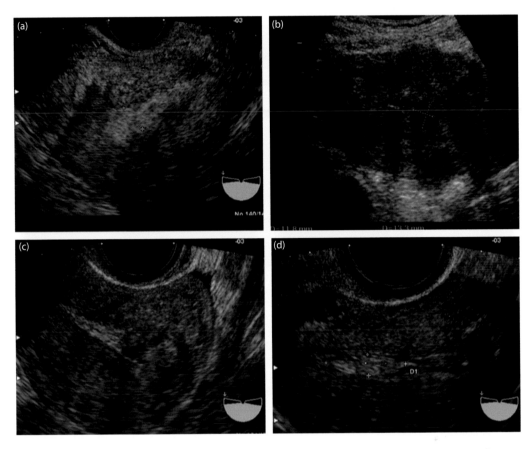

FIGURE 7.10 (a) Characteristic manifestation of adenomyosis; notice the diffusely asymmetrical myometrium, small cystic lesions, and irregular borders. (b) Transabdominal view of an enlarged uterus with numerous fibroids throughout the myometrium; indicative of diffuse leiomyomatosis. (c) Tiny submucosal fibroid—notice the round contour and hypoechogenicity. (d) Endometrial polyp—as opposed to a fibroid, polyps are "tongue shaped" and hyperechogenic. (From Clough A and Khalaf Y. Ultrasonography of uterine fibroids. In: Rizk B [ed] *Ultrasonography in Reproductive Medicine and Infertility.* Cambridge, UK: Cambridge University Press; 2010, pp. 88–96. With permission.)

Diffuse Uterine Leiomyomatosis

Diffuse uterine leiomyomatosis is an uncommon condition where there is widespread and consistent involvement of the whole myometrium by numerous fibroids (Figure 7.10b). SIS is also useful in differentiating diffuse endometrial changes from localized intracavitary lesions [24].

Endometrial Polyps

While fibroids arise from the myometrium, polyps are benign overgrowths of the endometrium that typically protrude into the uterine cavity [27]. The ultrasound appearance of the polyp is characteristically more hyperechoic than a fibroid, and it has a classic "tongue" shape, compared to the round form of a fibroid (Figure 7.10c and d). Not only is it challenging to differentiate a fibroid from a blood clot or a polyp, but fibroids can also obscure the endometrium on imaging or create the illusion of a thicker endometrial lining than there actually is [28]. TVS or color Doppler may be used initially to identify endometrial polyps, which may show up as hyperechoic aggregates enveloped by a hypoechoic endometrium [29]. While these methods may come with difficulty in distinguishing some polyps from diffusely thickened endometrium, SIS has the capability to make this distinction [30].

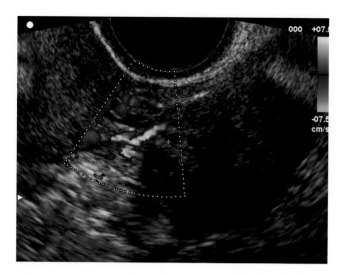

FIGURE 7.11   Color Doppler can identify the pedicle between a pedunculated fibroid and the uterus. (From Clough A and Khalaf Y. Ultrasonography of uterine fibroids. In: Rizk B [ed] *Ultrasonography in Reproductive Medicine and Infertility.* Cambridge, UK: Cambridge University Press; 2010, pp. 88–96. With permission.)

Ovarian Fibromas

Ovarian fibromas are benign tumors of stromal origin, and their classic appearance on ultrasound is of a spherical or elliptical solid tumor with acoustic shadows, even borders, and negligible vascularity on the periphery [31]. Using ultrasound, a pedunculated fibroid can be differentiated from an ovarian fibroma if both ovaries are identified separate from the fibroid. If the fibroid is of a substantial size, or is situated in the broad or round ligament, it might not be possible to detach it from the ovary. In this instance, it is imperative to use color Doppler to confidently pinpoint a pedicle connecting the fibroid to the uterus (Figure 7.11).

Leiomyosarcoma

A leiomyosarcoma is a rare, smooth muscle tumor that can appear similar to a large fibroid on ultrasound. Classically occurring in females in their mid-50s, the common symptoms include rapid growth, abnormal bleeding, and pain. Unfortunately, current imaging modalities have not been dependable in distinguishing between benign and malignant neoplasms [32]. A conclusive diagnosis can only be determined from a microscopic specimen.

Disseminated Peritoneal Leiomyomatosis

Disseminated peritoneal leiomyomatosis (DPL) is an unusual condition characterized by the manifestation of multifocal nodules and tumors that are composed of rapidly growing smooth muscle tissue spread throughout the peritoneum [33]. Although their dissemination suggests a metastatic process, the tumors are usually benign.

Proper Reporting of Ultrasound Findings

A suitable way to record fibroids that are found on ultrasound is to document their size and location, especially since these features are noteworthy in determining which treatment route to pursue [34]. Accurate measurement of fibroid size is important, as it has been shown to be useful in predicting the need for a major uterine procedure [35]. A great way to ensure accuracy in measurement is to measure the uterus and fibroids in three distinct perpendicular planes. They should each be measured at multiple time intervals throughout the ultrasound examination. It is crucial to measure fibroid size frequently, so as to establish how rapidly the fibroid is growing. Speed of growth can impact how the severity is discerned. The uterine location of each fibroid should then be recorded [36]. The location should be noted in two planes: first, in the transverse plane, and then in the longitudinal plane. If the fibroid is pedunculated, then documentation of the uterine origin and position in the pelvic cavity is required.

By following a logical order, physicians are more likely to convey valuable information in an effective manner. Utilizing standardized templates can help to further minimize confusion and mistakes. These, in turn, will help auditing procedures, which will pinpoint further areas for refinement. The suggested order for an ultrasound report is as follows: clinical history, area examined, description of findings, interpretation of findings, and conclusion. Regarding terminology, using equivocal terms such as "slightly" to describe an image are unhelpful to clinicians, as the connotation is often unclear. Doing so may mean subjecting patients to redundant further testing and imaging procedures [37]. A self-assured physician must be able to declare whether something definitely is, or is not, present in an image.

Conclusion

Overall, it is important to obtain decent preoperative imaging so that proper treatment can be provided. Without it, gynecologists are confronted with identifying the location and size of fibroids and the endometrium, which, in turn, can lead to uterine rupture during future pregnancies and higher risk of future myomectomies [38]. Proper treatment is also important in the patient with submucosal fibroids, which are shown to lower fertility rates [39]. Notably, studies have proven that by removing such fibroids, there is an improvement in both conception and live birth rates, including for those who undergo *in vitro* fertilization [40]. Future areas of research that might advance expertise in preoperative imaging include investigating fibroids in pregnant patients, as well as enhancing our ability to quickly differentiate fibroids versus sarcomas.

REFERENCES

1. Clough A and Khalaf Y. Ultrasonography of uterine fibroids. In: Rizk B (ed) *Ultrasonography in Reproductive Medicine and Infertility*. Cambridge, UK: Cambridge University Press; 2010, pp. 88–96.
2. Allahbadia GN and Merchant R. Ultrasound imaging of uterine fibroids: Evaluation and management. In: Rizk B and Puscheck E (eds) *Ultrasonography in Gynecology*. Cambridge, UK: Cambridge University Press; 2015, pp. 122–31.
3. Abuzeid MI and Joseph SK. Trans-vaginal ultrasound scan findings: Effect on treatment plan. In: Rizk B and Puscheck E (eds) *Ultrasonography in Gynecology*. Cambridge, UK: Cambridge University Press; 2015, pp. 80–93.
4. Mcwilliams M and Chennathukuzhi V. Recent advances in uterine fibroid etiology. *Semin Reprod Med*. 2017;35(02):181–9.
5. Williams AR. Uterine fibroids—What's new? *F1000Research*. 2017;6:2–6.
6. De La Cruz MD and Buchanan EM. Uterine fibroids: Diagnosis and treatment. *Am Fam Physician*. 2017;95(2):100–7. Accessed August 17, 2019. https://pdfs.semanticscholar.org/2d01/22a7aec04a18ca89f3b6e2d02c7ad53d1228.pdf
7. Liang B, Xie Y, Xu X, and Hu C. Diagnosis and treatment of submucous myoma of the uterus with interventional ultrasound. *Oncol Lett*. 2018;15:6189–94.
8. Eze C, Odumeru E, Ochie K, Nwadike U, and Agwuna K. Sonographic assessment of pregnancy co-existing with uterine leiomyoma in Owerri, Nigeria. *Afr Health Sci*. 2013;13(2):453–60.
9. Lucas VS, Burk RS, Creehan S, and Grap MJ. Utility of high-frequency ultrasound. *Plast Surg Nurs*. 2014;34(1):34–8.
10. Sharma K, Bora MK, Venkatesh B et al. Role of 3D ultrasound and Doppler in differentiating clinically suspected cases of leiomyoma and adenomyosis of uterus. *J Clin Diagn Res*. 2015;9(4):8–12.
11. Blaivas M. Chapter 22. Ultrasound evaluation of the pelvis. In: Belval B and Davis KJ (eds) *Critical Care Ultrasonography*. 2nd ed. New York, NY: McGraw-Hill Medical; 2013.

12. Klibanov AL and Hossack JA. Ultrasound in radiology: From anatomic, functional, molecular imaging to drug delivery and image-guided therapy. *Investig Radiol.* 2015;50(9):657–70.

13. El-Agwany A. Huge broad ligament fibroid with paracervical extension: A safe approach by same setting myomectomy before hysterectomy. *J Med Ultrasound.* 2018;26(1):45–7.

14. Van Den Bosch T, Ameye L, Van Schoubroeck D, Bourne T, and Timmerman D. Intra-cavitary uterine pathology in women with abnormal uterine bleeding: A prospective study of 1220 women. *Facts Views Vis OBGYN.* 2015;7(1):17–24. Accessed August 19, 2019. https://www.ncbi.nlm.nih.gov/pmc/articles/PMC4402439/

15. Donnez J and Dolmans M. Uterine fibroid management: From the present to the future. *Hum Reprod Update.* 2016;22(6):665–86.

16. Mavrelos D, Naftalin J, Hoo W, Ben-Nagi J, Holland T, and Jurkovic D. Preoperative assessment of submucous fibroids by three-dimensional saline contrast sonohysterography. *Ultrasound Obstet Gynecol.* 2011;38(3):350–4.

17. Laughlin-Tommaso SK, Hesley GK, Hopkins MR, Brandt KR, Zhu Y, and Stewart EA. Clinical limitations of the International Federation of Gynecology and Obstetrics (FIGO) classification of uterine fibroids. *Int J Gynecol Obstet.* 2017;139(2):143–8.

18. Marci R, Marcucci I, Marcucci AA et al. Hysterosalpingocontrast sonography (HyCoSy): Evaluation of the pain perception, side effects and complications. *BMC Med Imaging.* 2013;13(1):28.

19. Jinhe R. Color Doppler ultrasound in uterine arterial embolization. *Open Med.* 2017;12(1):489–93.

20. Krentel H, Cezar C, Becker S et al. From clinical symptoms to MR imaging: Diagnostic steps in adenomyosis. *BioMed Res Int.* 2017;2017:1–6.

21. Vu K, Fast AM, Shaffer RK et al. Evaluation of the routine use of pelvic MRI in women presenting with symptomatic uterine fibroids: When is pelvic MRI useful? *J Magn Reson Imaging.* 2019;49(7):271–81.

22. Maciel C, Tang YZ, Sahdev A, Madureira AM, and Morgado PV. Preprocedural MRI and MRA in planning fibroid embolization. *Diagn Interv Radiol.* 2017;23(2):163–71.

23. Woźniak A and Woźniak S. Ultrasonography of uterine leiomyomas. *Menopausal Rev.* 2017;16(4):113–7.

24. Khan A, Shehmar M, and Gupta J. Uterine fibroids: Current perspectives. *Int J Womens Health.* 2014;6:95–114.

25. Vannuccini S and Petraglia F. Recent advances in understanding and managing adenomyosis. *F1000Research.* 2019;8:1–10.

26. Li J, Chung JP, Wang S, Li T, and Duan H. The investigation and management of adenomyosis in women who wish to improve or preserve fertility. *BioMed Res Int.* 2018;2018(1):1–12.

27. Leyendecker G, Bilgicyildirim A, Inacker M et al. Adenomyosis and endometriosis. Re-visiting their association and further insights into the mechanisms of auto-traumatisation. An MRI study. *Arch Gynecol Obstet.* 2014;291(4):917–32.

28. Nijkang N P, Anderson L, Markham R, and Manconi F. Endometrial polyps: Pathogenesis, sequelae and treatment. *SAGE Open Med.* 2019;7:1–12.

29. Omari EA, Varghese, T, and Kliewer MA. A novel saline infusion sonohysterography-based strain imaging approach for evaluation of uterine abnormalities in vivo. *J Ultrasound Med.* 2012;31(4):609–15.

30. Kotdawala P, Kotdawala S, and Nagar N. Evaluation of endometrium in peri-menopausal abnormal uterine bleeding. *J Mid-Life Health.* 2013;4(1):16–21.

31. Sayasneh A, Ekechi C, Ferrara L et al. The characteristic ultrasound features of specific types of ovarian pathology (Review). *Int J Oncol.* 2014;46(2):445–58.

32. Chen I, Firth B, Hopkins L, Bougie O, Xie R, and Singh S. Clinical characteristics differentiating uterine sarcoma and fibroids. *JSLS.* 2018;22(1):1–6.

33. Ciebiera M, Słabuszewska-Jóźwiak A, Zaręba K, and Jakiel G. A case of disseminated peritoneal leiomyomatosis after two laparoscopic procedures due to uterine fibroids. *Wideochir Inne Tech Maloinwazyjne.* 2017;1:110–4.

34. Ahmad Zikri B, Sayed Aluwee S, Kato H et al. Magnetic resonance imaging of uterine fibroids: A preliminary investigation into the usefulness of 3D-rendered images for surgical planning. *SpringerPlus.* 2015;4(1):384–9.

35. Baird D, Saldana T, Shore D, Hill M, and Schectman J. A single baseline ultrasound assessment of fibroid presence and size is strongly predictive of future uterine procedure: 8-year follow-up of randomly sampled premenopausal women aged 35–49 years. *Hum Reprod.* 2015;30(12):2936–44.

36. Baird DD, Harmon QE, Upson K et al. A prospective, ultrasound-based study to evaluate risk factors for uterine fibroid incidence and growth: Methods and results of recruitment. *J Womens Health.* 2015;24(11):907–15.

37. Edwards H, Smith J, and Weston M. What makes a good ultrasound report? *Ultrasound.* 2013;22(1):57–60.

38. Kim YJ, Kim KG, Lee SR, Lee SH, and Kang BC. Preoperative 3-dimensional magnetic resonance imaging of uterine myoma and endometrium before myomectomy. *J Minim Invasive Gynecol.* 2017;24(2):309–14.

39. Purohit P and Vigneswaran K. Fibroids and infertility. *Curr Obstet Gynecol Rep.* 2016;5(2):81–8.

40. Guo XC and Segars JH. The impact and management of fibroids for fertility. *Obstet Gynecol Clin North Am.* 2012;39(4):521–33.

8

Fibroid Preoperative Imaging: Magnetic Resonance Imaging

Linda C. Chu, Mounes Aliyari Ghasabeh, and Ihab R. Kamel

CONTENTS

Introduction

Uterine leiomyomas, more commonly known as fibroids, are benign neoplasms composed of smooth muscle and fibrous connective tissue [1]. They are the most common gynecologic neoplasm, with prevalence of 70%–80% of women by 50 years of age [2]. The prevalence of uterine leiomyomas increases with age [2–5] and is higher for African American women [2–5]. Many women with uterine leiomyomas are asymptomatic, and these leiomyomas are incidentally found on physical examination or imaging [2]. However, leiomyomas can cause significant morbidity including dysfunctional uterine bleeding, iron deficiency anemia, pelvic pain and pressure, and infertility [6].

Although ultrasonography (US) is the preferred initial imaging test for patients with suspected uterine leiomyomas, magnetic resonance imaging (MRI) is the most accurate imaging modality for the detection and localization of leiomyomas. MRI has superior tissue contrast resolution compared to US, which is important in localization and classification of leiomyomas. MRI can also be used to diagnose alternative and/or coexisting pelvic pathology. Therefore, MRI is the imaging modality of choice in determining the best treatment options and preoperative planning. This chapter reviews the application of MRI in preoperative imaging of uterine leiomyomas.

Magnetic Resonance Imaging Techniques

Pelvic MRI is performed with a standard phased-array surface coil. At our institution, our protocol includes a T2-weighted sequence in the sagittal and axial plane, a three-dimensional (3D) T2-weighted sequence, axial T1-weighted fast spin echo, axial diffusion weighted sequence, and dynamic fat-suppressed pre- and postcontrast gradient echo sequence in the axial and sagittal planes. T2-weighted images are essential for anatomic delineation of the uterine leiomyoma and its relationship to the endometrium, myometrium, and serosal surface. The 3D T2-weighted sequence allows for multiplanar reconstruction and can be helpful for anatomic delineation as the uterus may be positioned obliquely within the pelvis. The T1-weighted images with and without fat saturation are useful to differentiate between fat and blood products in the characterization of any coexisting adnexal pathology. Pre- and postcontrast images with fat suppression are used to determine enhancement of the leiomyomas, which is important in predicting treatment response to uterine artery embolization (UAE). An optional MR angiography can be included to facilitate the visualization of blood supply of the leiomyomas and may be helpful for UAE planning.

Magnetic Resonance Imaging Features of Uterine Leiomyomas and Differential Diagnosis

Uterine leiomyomas classically appear as well-circumscribed masses that are T2 hypointense relative to the outer myometrium. Contrast enhancement may vary and can be homogeneous, heterogeneous, or minimal (Figure 8.1) [7,8]. Uterine leiomyomas can occasionally undergo degeneration and present with atypical imaging features. Uterine leiomyomas with hyaline degeneration contain internal T2 hypointense foci due to the presence of dystrophic calcifications. The presence of cystic or myxoid degeneration results in T2 hyperintense signal without associated contrast enhancement (Figure 8.2) [7,9,10]. Red degeneration refers to hemorrhagic infarction and is associated with pregnancy and oral contraceptives. These leiomyomas demonstrate diffuse or peripheral rim T1 hyperintensity (Figure 8.3) [11].

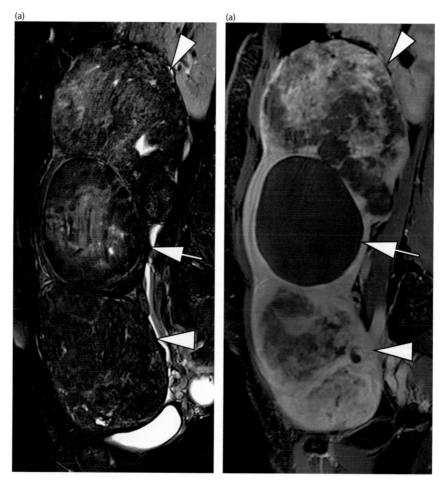

FIGURE 8.1 A 41-year-old woman with history of abdominal mass. (a) Sagittal T2-weighted magnetic resonance (MR) image of the abdomen and pelvis shows a large fibroid uterus with intramural leiomyoma (FIGO type 4, arrow) and subserosal leiomyomas (FIGO type 5, arrowheads). (b) Sagittal T1-weighted postcontrast MR image of the abdomen and pelvis shows absence of enhancement of the intramural leiomyoma (arrow) and heterogeneous enhancement of the subserosal leiomyomas (arrowheads).

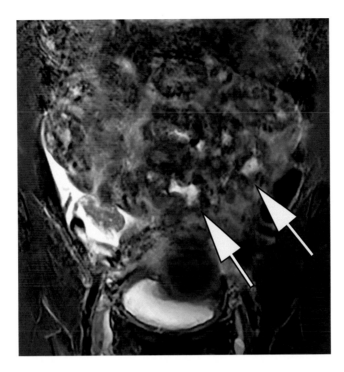

FIGURE 8.2 A 42-year-old woman with history of uterine fibroids. Multiple degenerated fibroids were noted on hysterectomy specimen. Coronal T2-weighted magnetic resonance image shows an enlarged uterus with numerous predominantly T2 hypointense masses with central T2 hyperintense signal (arrows), compatible with degenerated leiomyomas.

Differential diagnosis for uterine leiomyoma includes leiomyosarcoma and adenomyosis. Uterine leiomyosarcomas are rare and are found in 0.23%–0.49% of patients who underwent myomectomy or hysterectomy for presumptive diagnosis of uterine leiomyomas [12,13]. The prevalence of leiomyosarcoma increases with age and can be found in up to 1.7% of hysterectomy specimens [13]. Most uterine leiomyosarcomas are believed to arise *de novo* from uterine myometrium or connective tissue surrounding the uterine vasculature. Malignant transformation of preexisting uterine leiomyomas has been reported [14]. A number of imaging features have been described to differentiate leiomyosarcomas from leiomyomas, including large tumor size, invasive features, rapid growth especially in postmenopausal women, T2 hyperintensity, T1 hyperintensity (hemorrhage), low apparent diffusion coefficient (ADC) (high tumor cellularity), nodular borders, and inhomogeneous enhancement with central necrosis (Figure 8.4) [7,14–18]. However, due to the rarity of leiomyosarcomas compared to leiomyomas, a myometrial mass demonstrating "suspicious" features is still more likely to represent an atypical leiomyoma rather than leiomyosarcoma. Currently, there is no imaging technique that can reliably differentiate leiomyosarcoma from leiomyoma [6,14,15].

Differential diagnosis of leiomyoma also includes adenomyosis, which is characterized by extension of ectopic endometrial glands and stroma into the myometrium with adjacent myometrial hypertrophy [19–21]. The estimated prevalence of adenomyosis ranges from 14% to 66% depending on the study population [21]. Adenomyosis can result in diffuse thickening of the junctional zone, or it can present as a more focal T2 hypointense mass inseparable from the junctional zone (Figure 8.5) [20]. The ill-defined borders and contiguity with the junctional zone are helpful in distinguishing adenomyosis from leiomyoma.

Classification of Uterine Leiomyomas and Implications for Management

The clinical presentation of uterine leiomyomas is variable, depending on size, number, and location of these leiomyomas. Leiomyomas are classified as submucosal, intramural, and subserosal based on their relationship to the endometrium and external contour of the uterus. Heavy menstrual bleeding and

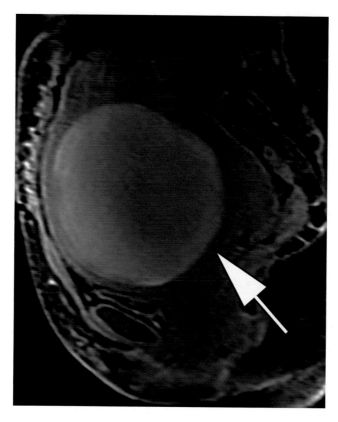

FIGURE 8.3   A 40-year-old woman with history of uterine fibroid. Sagittal T1-weighted fat-suppressed precontrast image shows an intrinsically T1 hyperintense myometrial mass (arrow), compatible with red degeneration of uterine leiomyoma with hemorrhage.

painful periods are the most frequent symptoms and can be caused by submucosal leiomyomas that distort the uterine cavity [22] and large intramural fibroids [23]. Bulk symptoms could be related to size, and usually occur with subserosal, pedunculated, and large intramural leiomyomas [24]. The negative effects of leiomyomas on pregnancy are determined by both location and size. Submucosal and large (greater than 5 cm) intramural leiomyomas have the strongest risk for decreased implantation and higher risk of spontaneous abortion [25,26].

Asymptomatic leiomyomas do not require any treatment. Treatment approaches for symptomatic leiomyomas depend on accurate localization and pretreatment mapping. MRI has been shown to be superior to ultrasound in pretreatment mapping, especially in patients with larger uteri or in patients with multiple leiomyomas [27]. MRI is also more consistent in the detection of uterine cavity abnormalities and submucosal components compared to US [28]. However, there remains significant variability in what criteria radiologists use for leiomyoma localization and how they report these findings. In 2011, the International Federation of Gynecology and Obstetrics (FIGO) proposed a classification system to standardize the reporting for causes of abnormal uterine bleeding. It includes a leiomyoma subclassification system (Table 8.1) that distinguishes submucosal leiomyomas from others, as the former are more likely to be associated with abnormal uterine bleeding [29,30]. Submucosal leiomyomas are divided into three types: pedunculated intracavitary (type 0), submucosal leiomyoma with less than 50% intramural involvement (type 1), and submucosal leiomyoma with 50% or greater intramural involvement (type 2) (Figures 8.6 and 8.7). The other leiomyomas include intramural, subserosal, cervical, and parasitic leiomyomas. Type 3 refers to a leiomyoma that is 100% intramural but contacts the endometrium (Figure 8.7). A type 4 leiomyoma is entirely intramural (Figure 8.1). Type 5 and 6 leiomyomas refer to subserosal leiomyomas with 50% or greater intramural involvement and less than 50% intramural involvement, respectively

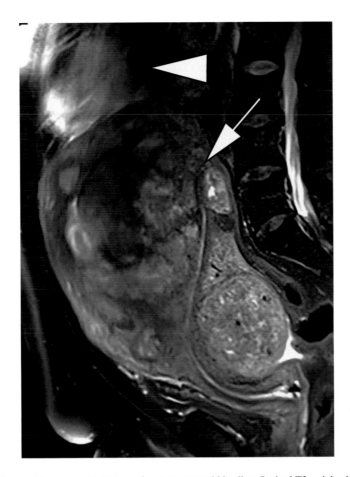

FIGURE 8.4 A 54-year-old woman with history of postmenopausal bleeding. Sagittal T2-weighted magnetic resonance image shows an enlarged uterus replaced by numerous heterogeneous masses. There is a dominant intramural mass with heterogeneous T2 signal in the anterior uterine body (arrow) and a pedunculated subserosal T2 hyperintense mass at the fundus (arrowhead). Patient underwent hysterectomy, which demonstrated uterine leiomyosarcoma.

(Figures 8.1 and 8.7). Type 7 refers to subserosal pedunculated leiomyoma, and type 8 is reserved for leiomyomas that do not relate to the myometrium, such as cervical or parasitic leiomyomas. Hybrid leiomyomas with less than 50% submucosal and less than 50% subserosal involvement are designated type 2-5 (Figure 8.8) [29,30].

Preoperative MRI with standardized reporting and classification of leiomyomas allows for optimal selection of surgical approach and preoperative planning (Table 8.2). The MRI report should provide the overall size of the uterus and an approximate number of leiomyomas. The report should provide detailed description of dominant leiomyomas with and without submucosal components, as this localization is key for selection of the treatment approach. The degree of contrast enhancement should be included, as it is an important factor in preoperative planning for UAE. Any aggressive features or coexisting pelvic pathology (e.g., adenomyosis, adnexal mass) should also be included.

Hysterectomy is the most definitive treatment for management of uterine leiomyomas. Myomectomy, UAE, and MR-guided focused ultrasound are alternatives to hysterectomy [6,31]. Myomectomy can be performed with hysteroscopic, laparoscopic, and open approaches depending on the size, number, and location of leiomyomas. Hysteroscopic myomectomy should be considered the first-line conservative surgical treatment for intracavitary leiomyoma (type 0). Submucosal leiomyomas (type 0, 1, and 2) up to 4 to 5 cm in diameter can be removed hysteroscopically by experienced surgeons [6,31].

UAE is an alternative conservative therapy for treatment of symptomatic leiomyomas. There are MRI features in addition to size and location that are important in appropriate patient selection and

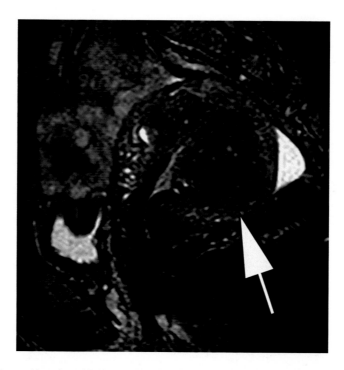

FIGURE 8.5 A 45-year-old woman with history of pelvic pain. Sagittal T2-weighted magnetic resonance image of the pelvis shows thickening of the posterior junctional zone without discrete borders, compatible with adenomyosis (arrow).

TABLE 8.1

International Federation of Gynecology and Obstetrics (FIGO) Classification of Uterine Leiomyomas

Classification	Type	Criteria
SM—Submucosal	0	Pedunculated intracavitary
	1	Less than 50% intramural
	2	50% or greater intramural
O—Other	3	Contacts endometrium; 100% intramural
	4	Intramural
	5	Subserosal 50% or greater intramural
	6	Subserosal less than 50% intramural
	7	Subserosal pedunculated
	8	Other (specify, e.g., cervical, parasitic)
Hybrid leiomyomas (impact both endometrium and serosa)	2-5	Submucosal and subserosal, each with less than half the diameter in the endometrial and peritoneal cavities, respectively

Source: Table adapted from Munro MG, Critchley HO, Broder MS, Fraser IS; FIGO Working Group on Menstrual Disorders. *Int J Gynaecol Obstet.* 2011;113(1):3–13; Munro MG, Critchley HO, Fraser IS; FIGO Menstrual Disorders Working Group. *Fertil Steril.* 2011;95(7):2204–8, 8.e1–3.

preoperative planning. The degree of contrast enhancement is an important factor in predicting success of UAE. Leiomyomas that do not enhance on preoperative imaging (Figure 8.1) are already devascularized and are less likely to respond to treatment [38,39]. Cervical leiomyomas have an alternative blood supply and may not become devascularized after UAE [40]. Patients with these leiomyomas may not benefit from UAE, and alternative treatment approaches should be considered.

UAE was traditionally thought to be contraindicated in patients with pedunculated subserosal leiomyomas due to the potential risk of stalk necrosis and detachment. A number of studies have shown no increased complication rates in patients undergoing UAE for pedunculated subserosal leiomyomas

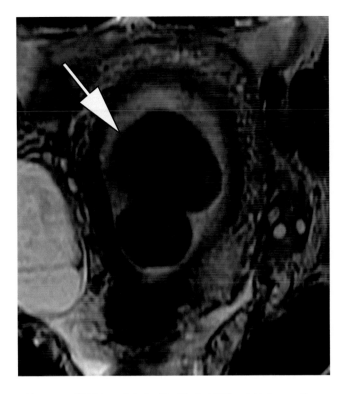

FIGURE 8.6 A 29-year-old woman with history of uterine fibroids. Axial T2-weighted magnetic resonance image of the pelvis shows a lobulated T2 hypointense mass within the endometrial cavity, consistent with an intracavity leiomyoma (FIGO type 0).

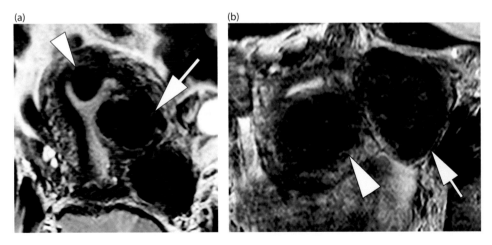

FIGURE 8.7 A 44-year-old woman with history of uterine fibroids. (a) Coronal T2-weighted magnetic resonance (MR) image of the pelvis shows two submucosal leiomyomas. One leiomyoma has less than 50% intramural component (FIGO type 1, arrowhead), and the other leiomyoma has 50% or greater intramural component (FIGO type 2, arrow). (b) Axial T2-weighted MR image of the pelvis at the level of the fundus shows additional leiomyomas. There is one intramural leiomyoma with endometrial contact (FIGO type 3, arrowhead) and a subserosal leiomyoma with less than 50% intramural component (FIGO type 6, arrow).

[32–34]. However, it is helpful to include measurement of the stalk diameter of pedunculated subserosal leiomyomas [35] so that the interventionalist can counsel the patients appropriately. Submucosal leiomyomas can become intracavitary following UAE, and this has been observed in up to 50% of cases [36]. The risk can be assessed on preoperative MRI by the size of the endometrial interface relative to the size of the leiomyoma [37].

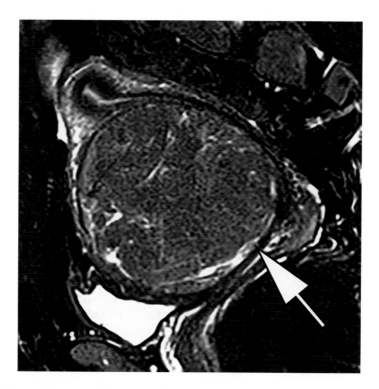

FIGURE 8.8   A 35-year-old woman with history of dysfunctional uterine bleeding. Sagittal T2-weighted magnetic resonance image of the pelvis shows an intramural leiomyoma with both submucosal and subserosal components (FIGO type 2-5, arrow).

TABLE 8.2

Proposed Magnetic Resonance Reporting Template for Uterine Leiomyoma

Findings:
Uterus: Measures _____ cm
Number of uterus fibroids: ___
Dominant fibroids without submucosal component:
1. ___ cm [FIGO type] fibroid in the [location] with [no, minimal, moderate, or marked] contrast enhancement. [Include any aggressive features]
Dominant fibroids with submucosal component:
1. ___ cm [FIGO type] fibroid in the [location] with [no, minimal, moderate, or marked] contrast enhancement. Approximately ___% submucosal component. [Include any aggressive features]
Endometrium: Measures ___ mm
Junctional zone: Measures __ mm
Cervix:
Vagina:
Ovaries:
Other:

Conclusion

MRI is the modality of choice for preoperative planning of uterine leiomyomas, as it is superior to ultrasound in the depiction of the number, size, and location of leiomyomas. A standardized classification and reporting system provides important information in selecting the most appropriate treatment approach and predicting treatment success.

REFERENCES

1. Prayson RA and Hart WR. Pathologic considerations of uterine smooth muscle tumors. *Obstet Gynecol Clin North Am*. 1995;22(4):637–57.
2. Baird DD, Dunson DB, Hill MC, Cousins D, and Schectman JM. High cumulative incidence of uterine leiomyoma in black and white women: Ultrasound evidence. *Am J Obstet Gynecol*. 2003;188(1):100–7.
3. Borgfeldt C and Andolf E. Transvaginal ultrasonographic findings in the uterus and the endometrium: Low prevalence of leiomyoma in a random sample of women age 25–40 years. *Acta Obstet Gynecol Scand*. 2000;79(3):202–7.
4. Marshall LM, Spiegelman D, Barbieri RL et al. Variation in the incidence of uterine leiomyoma among premenopausal women by age and race. *Obstet Gynecol*. 1997;90(6):967–73.
5. Stewart EA, Cookson CL, Gandolfo RA, and Schulze-Rath R. Epidemiology of uterine fibroids: A systematic review. *BJOG*. 2017;124(10):1501–12.
6. Vilos GA, Allaire C, Laberge PY et al. The management of uterine leiomyomas. *J Obstet Gynaecol Can*. 2015;37(2):157–78.
7. Murase E, Siegelman ES, Outwater EK, Perez-Jaffe LA, and Tureck RW. Uterine leiomyomas: Histopathologic features, MR imaging findings, differential diagnosis, and treatment. *Radiographics*. 1999;19(5):1179–97.
8. Hricak H, Tscholakoff D, Heinrichs L et al. Uterine leiomyomas: Correlation of MR, histopathologic findings, and symptoms. *Radiology*. 1986;158(2):385–91.
9. Okizuka H, Sugimura K, Takemori M, Obayashi C, Kitao M, and Ishida T. MR detection of degenerating uterine leiomyomas. *J Comput Assist Tomogr*. 1993;17(5):760–6.
10. Bolan C and Caserta MP. MR imaging of atypical fibroids. *Abdom Radiol (NY)*. 2016;41(12):2332–49.
11. Nakai G, Yamada T, Hamada T et al. Pathological findings of uterine tumors preoperatively diagnosed as red degeneration of leiomyoma by MRI. *Abdom Radiol (NY)*. 2017;42(7):1825–31.
12. Parker WH, Fu YS, and Berek JS. Uterine sarcoma in patients operated on for presumed leiomyoma and rapidly growing leiomyoma. *Obstet Gynecol*. 1994;83(3):414–8.
13. Leibsohn S, d'Ablaing G, Mishell DR, and Schlaerth JB. Leiomyosarcoma in a series of hysterectomies performed for presumed uterine leiomyomas. *Am J Obstet Gynecol*. 1990;162(4):968–74; discussion 74–6.
14. Kaganov H, Ades A, and Fraser DS. Preoperative magnetic resonance imaging diagnostic features of uterine leiomyosarcomas: A systematic review. *Int J Technol Assess Health Care*. 2018;34(2):172–9.
15. Kubik-Huch RA, Weston M, Nougaret S et al. European Society of Urogenital Radiology (ESUR) Guidelines: MR imaging of leiomyomas. *Eur Radiol*. 2018;28(8):3125–37.
16. Lakhman Y, Veeraraghavan H, Chaim J et al. Differentiation of uterine leiomyosarcoma from atypical leiomyoma: Diagnostic accuracy of qualitative MR imaging features and feasibility of texture analysis. *Eur Radiol*. 2017;27(7):2903–15.
17. Tanaka YO, Nishida M, Tsunoda H, Okamoto Y, and Yoshikawa H. Smooth muscle tumors of uncertain malignant potential and leiomyosarcomas of the uterus: MR findings. *J Magn Reson Imaging*. 2004;20(6):998–1007.
18. Goto A, Takeuchi S, Sugimura K, and Maruo T. Usefulness of Gd-DTPA contrast-enhanced dynamic MRI and serum determination of LDH and its isozymes in the differential diagnosis of leiomyosarcoma from degenerated leiomyoma of the uterus. *Int J Gynecol Cancer*. 2002;12(4):354–61.
19. Sudderuddin S, Helbren E, Telesca M, Williamson R, and Rockall A. MRI appearances of benign uterine disease. *Clin Radiol*. 2014;69(11):1095–104.
20. Outwater EK, Siegelman ES, and Van Deerlin V. Adenomyosis: Current concepts and imaging considerations. *AJR Am J Roentgenol*. 1998;170(2):437–41.
21. Vercellini P, Viganò P, Somigliana E, Daguati R, Abbiati A, and Fedele L. Adenomyosis: Epidemiological factors. *Best Pract Res Clin Obstet Gynaecol*. 2006;20(4):465–77.
22. Puri K, Famuyide AO, Erwin PJ, Stewart EA, and Laughlin-Tommaso SK. Submucosal fibroids and the relation to heavy menstrual bleeding and anemia. *Am J Obstet Gynecol*. 2014;210(1):38.e1–7.
23. Wegienka G, Baird DD, Hertz-Picciotto I et al. Self-reported heavy bleeding associated with uterine leiomyomata. *Obstet Gynecol*. 2003;101(3):431–7.
24. Wu CQ, Lefebvre G, Frecker H, and Husslein H. Urinary retention and uterine leiomyomas: A case series and systematic review of the literature. *Int Urogynecol J*. 2015;26(9):1277–84.

25. Oliveira FG, Abdelmassih VG, Diamond MP, Dozortsev D, Melo NR, and Abdelmassih R. Impact of subserosal and intramural uterine fibroids that do not distort the endometrial cavity on the outcome of in vitro fertilization-intracytoplasmic sperm injection. *Fertil Steril.* 2004;81(3):582–7.

26. Laughlin-Tommaso SK. Alternatives to hysterectomy: Management of uterine fibroids. *Obstet Gynecol Clin North Am.* 2016;43(3):397–413.

27. Dueholm M, Lundorf E, Hansen ES, Ledertoug S, and Olesen F. Accuracy of magnetic resonance imaging and transvaginal ultrasonography in the diagnosis, mapping, and measurement of uterine myomas. *Am J Obstet Gynecol.* 2002;186(3):409–15.

28. Dueholm M, Lundorf E, Sørensen JS, Ledertoug S, Olesen F, and Laursen H. Reproducibility of evaluation of the uterus by transvaginal sonography, hysterosonographic examination, hysteroscopy and magnetic resonance imaging. *Hum Reprod.* 2002;17(1):195–200.

29. Munro MG, Critchley HO, Broder MS, Fraser IS; FIGO Working Group on Menstrual Disorders. FIGO classification system (PALM-COEIN) for causes of abnormal uterine bleeding in nongravid women of reproductive age. *Int J Gynaecol Obstet.* 2011;113(1):3–13.

30. Munro MG, Critchley HO, Fraser IS; FIGO Menstrual Disorders Working Group. The FIGO classification of causes of abnormal uterine bleeding in the reproductive years. *Fertil Steril.* 2011;95(7):2204–8, 8.e1–3.

31. American College of Obstetricians and Gynecologists. ACOG practice bulletin. Alternatives to hysterectomy in the management of leiomyomas. *Obstet Gynecol.* 2008;112(2 Pt 1):387–400.

32. Margau R, Simons ME, Rajan DK et al. Outcomes after uterine artery embolization for pedunculated subserosal leiomyomas. *J Vasc Interv Radiol.* 2008;19(5):657–61.

33. Smeets AJ, Nijenhuis RJ, Boekkooi PF et al. Safety and effectiveness of uterine artery embolization in patients with pedunculated fibroids. *J Vasc Interv Radiol.* 2009;20(9):1172–5.

34. Kim YS, Han K, Kim MD et al. Uterine artery embolization for pedunculated subserosal leiomyomas: Evidence of safety and efficacy. *J Vasc Interv Radiol.* 2018;29(4):497–501.

35. Deshmukh SP, Gonsalves CF, Guglielmo FF, and Mitchell DG. Role of MR imaging of uterine leiomyomas before and after embolization. *Radiographics.* 2012;32(6):E251–81.

36. Radeleff B, Eiers M, Bellemann N et al. Expulsion of dominant submucosal fibroids after uterine artery embolization. *Eur J Radiol.* 2010;75(1):e57–63.

37. Verma SK, Bergin D, Gonsalves CF, Mitchell DG, Lev-Toaff AS, and Parker L. Submucosal fibroids becoming endocavitary following uterine artery embolization: Risk assessment by MRI. *AJR Am J Roentgenol.* 2008;190(5):1220–6.

38. Nikolaidis P, Siddiqi AJ, Carr JC et al. Incidence of nonviable leiomyomas on contrast material-enhanced pelvic MR imaging in patients referred for uterine artery embolization. *J Vasc Interv Radiol.* 2005;16(11):1465–71.

39. Harman M, Zeteroğlu S, Arslan H, Sengül M, and Etlik O. Predictive value of magnetic resonance imaging signal and contrast-enhancement characteristics on post-embolization volume reduction of uterine fibroids. *Acta Radiol.* 2006;47(4):427–35.

40. Kim MD, Lee M, Jung DC et al. Limited efficacy of uterine artery embolization for cervical leiomyomas. *J Vasc Interv Radiol.* 2012;23(2):236–40.

9

Interventional Procedures

Kristin Patzkowsky

CONTENTS

Introduction

Alternative procedural treatments, such as uterine artery embolization (UAE), magnetic resonance–guided focused ultrasound (MRgFUS), and radiofrequency ablation (RFA), can be excellent options for patients who would like to avoid major surgery, those who are poor surgical candidates, and/or those who would like to keep their uterus while treating their fibroids. Each procedure is associated with positive outcomes in the appropriately selected patient. As with any intervention, there are ideal candidates for each procedure based on fibroid burden and fibroid characteristics. Every patient is unique in terms of fibroid burden, her symptoms, and treatment goals. These factors must be carefully considered when counseling your patient about realistic treatment outcomes and expectations. It is important to note that the desire for future childbearing is a relative contraindication to each of these interventions.

UAE was first described for the treatment of fibroids in 1995 and since then has been popularly and widely used. Many scientific studies on UAE have been published. Relative to UAE, RFA and MRgFUS are still in their infancy, and the scientific studies are not nearly as robust.

Uterine Artery Embolization

UAE, sometimes referred to as uterine fibroid embolization (UFE), is a procedure typically performed by interventional radiology or vascular surgery. A permanent occlusive agent is used to block the uterine arteries and/or individual branches feeding a fibroid(s). Normal uterine tissue recovers from the ischemic insult because of accessory blood flow to the uterus, but fibroids are preferentially affected leading to irreversible ischemic injury, necrosis, and ultimately a permanent reduction in fibroid size.

Procedure Specifics

Patients are given local anesthesia or light conscious sedation while arterial access is obtained, most commonly via the femoral artery at the groin or radial artery at the wrist. A catheter is threaded back through the arterial access point to the uterine artery under fluoroscopic guidance. Once there, polyvinyl alcohol (PVA) particles measuring 200–500 microns are placed until complete occlusion of the artery feeding the fibroid(s) is verified. PVA particles are the most commonly used embolic agent, but other agents can be used with equivalent efficacy including tris-acryl gelatin or polyzene-F hydrogel microspheres [1]. The procedure takes approximately 1 hour to complete and is commonly performed as an outpatient procedure, though an initial overnight stay for pain control may be required. Pain medications are required for an average of 4–7 days, and most patients resume usual activities within 1–2 weeks.

Short-Term Outcomes

The Ontario Uterine Artery Embolization trial was a prospective single-arm trial where UAE was performed in 538 women by 11 interventional radiologists at 8 centers in Ontario, Canada [2,3]. Preprocedure symptoms included menorrhagia, pelvic pain, and bulk symptoms. The average age of the participant was 43 years (range of 19–56 years), and 30% wished to retain their fertility. Bilateral UAE was successful in 97% of cases. Unilateral UAE was performed in 14 cases (2.5%), and UAE was unsuccessful in 3 (0.5%) participants. The average procedure time was 61 minutes. Three-month telephone interviews were completed in 96%, and 3-month post-UAE ultrasounds were available in 86% of cases. At 3 months, there was a 35% median uterine volume reduction and a 42% dominant fibroid reduction. There was a self-reported reduction in mean menstrual duration from 7.6 to 5.4 days, and median pad count per day had significantly decreased. Patients also reported improvement in menorrhagia (83% of patients reporting improved), dysmenorrhea (77%), and urinary frequency/urgency (86%). At 3 months' postprocedure, 91% reported satisfaction with the procedure.

Long-Term Outcomes and Reintervention

A Cochrane database review for UAE reported a decrease in fibroid size ranging from 30% to 46% [4]. The longest UAE follow-up study to date is the EMMY trial with a 10-year follow-up [5]. This study included 28 Dutch hospitals, and women who were eligible for hysterectomy for symptomatic fibroids were randomized to UAE versus hysterectomy. Included were 177 patients: 89 randomized to UAE and 88 to hysterectomy. The mean duration of follow-up was 133 months, and the mean patient age was 57 years. There was an 84% response rate. Thirty-five percent had secondary hysterectomy, though only 31% if successful UAE was included. Health-related quality of life improved in both groups and remained stable over time, with 78% in the UAE group and 87% in the hysterectomy group reporting being very satisfied.

At 2 years, 60%–80% of patients reported an improvement in heavy menstrual bleeding, and 77%–85% of patients reported an improvement in dysmenorrhea [3,6]. Bulk-related symptoms are not as well studied. In the EMMY trial, there were comparable rates of improvement in bulk-related symptoms in the UAE and hysterectomy groups at 2 years, though other studies have not shown significant improvement in bulk-related symptoms [6–8].

Reintervention rates vary depending on the length of follow-up and initial patient characteristics. In the EMMY trial at 5- and 10-year follow-up, approximately 30% of patients underwent secondary hysterectomy. A meta-analysis of four randomized controlled trials found a similar number at 5-year follow-up [9]. Those with larger uteri and greater fibroid burden at baseline are at higher risk of failure [10,11]. Unilateral embolization, which occurs in approximately 5% of patients, is consistently seen as a risk factor for failure. Factors predictive of unilateral embolization include anatomical differences, arterial spasm, and preoperative gonadotropin-releasing hormone (GnRH) agonist use.

Risks

Postprocedural pain appears to increase with the volume of fibroid embolized. Up to 10% of patients may require readmission for pain control [9]. Postembolization syndrome is seen in approximately 10% of patients undergoing UAE and is characterized by fever, leukocytosis, pain, nausea, and fatigue [9]. Symptoms are usually mild and self-limited and are managed with supportive care. Endometrial infection more commonly occurs (0.5%) after embolization of a submucosal fibroid. Up to 20% of patients will report vaginal discharge that can last for up to 6 months after the procedure [12]. Ovarian failure is directly related to age at time of procedure and is more likely to occur with age older than 45 years. Other rare but serious complications can occur, such as uterine necrosis, sepsis secondary to necrotic fibroid, necrosis of unintended target (lower limbs, gluteus) via migration of embolic particles, or pulmonary embolus [13–15].

Pregnancy Afterward

Pregnancy outcomes post-UAE have largely been described in case reports and observational studies. A meta-analysis from 2010 by Homer and Saridogan detailed the outcomes of 227 pregnancies after UAE compared to fibroid-containing pregnancies matched for age and fibroid location [16]. There was a 35% miscarriage rate in the UAE pregnancies compared to 16% in the fibroid-containing pregnancies (odds ratio [OR] 2.8; 95% confidence interval [CI] 2.0–3.8). UAE pregnancies were more likely to be delivery by cesarean section (66% versus 48.5% OR 2.1; 95% CI 1.4–2.9) and experience postpartum hemorrhage (13.9% versus 2.5%; OR 6.4; 95% CI 3.5–11.7). There did not appear to be a difference on preterm delivery, intrauterine growth restriction, or malpresentation. Further studies are needed to detect a statistical difference in obstetric outcomes.

Magnetic Resonance–Guided Focused Ultrasound

MRgFUS is a procedure performed by interventional radiology and treats fibroids by way of thermal necrosis. MRgFUS is able to target fibroids individually as opposed to the entire uterus as with UAE. One recognized benefit of directed fibroid treatment is that there is no effect on ovarian tissue and no risk of ovarian failure. Conversely, if each fibroid must be treated individually, there are natural limits to fibroid size and number than can be reasonably approached via this method, and the procedure can be lengthy.

MRgFUS was approved by the U.S. Food and Drug Administration for use in the United States in 2004. This procedure has not achieved the same level of popularity as UAE, likely secondary to multiple factors including narrow selection criteria, lengthy procedure, and cost.

Procedure Specifics

The patient is given intravenous (IV) conscious sedation while lying prone on the specialized MRgFUS table (e.g., ExAblate [InSightec, Haifa, Israel]). This table has an ultrasound transducer (frequency range 1–1.5 MHz) built into the MR machine. Because ultrasound waves do not pass through air, the abdomen is submerged in water, or an ultrasound gel pad is placed between the patient and the transducer. Magnetic resonance imaging (MRI) is used to visualize the fibroids and surrounding structures. A phased-array transducer delivers ultrasound pulses of thermal energy to a specified point, termed a *sonication*. MRI gives real-time thermal feedback so the operator can adjust the power to achieve the desired tissue effect, generally 65°C–85°C to achieve coagulative necrosis. Each sonication area is approximately 0.5 cm^3, roughly the size of a bean. Thus, multiple sonications or more than one treatment session are required to treat a single fibroid. Several studies support a mean procedure length of 3–4 hours [17–19]. Preprocedure treatment with a GnRH-agonist to decrease fibroid size is an effective means of reducing the number of sonications necessary and may also augment treatment effect in certain types of fibroids [20,21]. After treatment, MRI with IV gadolinium is performed to assess the amount of tissue devascularization. This is measured as the nonperfused volume (NPV), that is, the volume of tissue where blood flow is cut off after treatment, as a change from the baseline exam. The greater the NPV, the greater is the region of induced necrosis as compared to baseline. Not surprisingly, the effectiveness of MRgFUS has been shown to be related to the NPV achieved.

Short-Term Outcomes

As previously mentioned, the NPV ratio is directly linked to efficacy, as is the pretreatment signal intensity. Fibroids are commonly classified into type 1, 2, or 3 fibroids based on the signal intensity of pretreatment T2-weighted images, where type 1 has a low-intensity image comparable to skeletal muscle, type 2 has an intensity lower than myometrium but higher than skeletal muscle, and type 3 has an image intensity higher than or equal to the surrounding myometrium. Type 3 fibroids are least responsive to MRgFUS, likely secondary to increased cell density [17–19].

The greatest change in fibroid size and symptom relief occurs in the first 3 months after the procedure [17,19]. In a study by Funaki et al., 91 Japanese women were followed for 24 months after MRgFUS by symptoms severity score and repeat imaging. At 6 months after the procedure, type 1 and 2 myomas decreased an average of −36.5% and −39.5% at 24 months. Type 3 myomas did not show a reduction in size at 6 months ($-9.1 \pm 44.8\%$, $n = 9$).

The study by Stewart et al. focused on symptom severity of quality of life measures. At 6 and 12 months after the procedure, 71% and 51% of participants met the targeted efficacy in quality of life measures. Similarly, symptom severity scores improved with a 39% and 36% reduction at 6- and 12-month time points.

Long-Term Outcomes and Reintervention

Long-term outcomes and reintervention rates vary widely between studies, though this is not surprising given the disparate outcomes depending on volume of fibroid treated, NPV%, and fibroid signal intensity. At 2 years, Fuanki et al. reported a 14% reintervention rate for type 1 and 2 fibroids and a 22% reintervention rate for type 3 fibroids.

The 2007 study by Stewart et al. exemplified the impact of the NPV ratio on clinical outcomes, where the high NPV group had a greater improvement in symptom severity score that persisted up to 24 months [22]. There was also a statistically significant difference in the number of women undergoing additional treatment in the high versus low NPV, where an increased NPV reduces the risk of undergoing additional leiomyoma treatment.

A cohort study published in 2014 by Quinn et al. followed 280 women for up to 5 years after MRgFUS [21]. There was a 75% response rate from 239 women who had the procedure at least 3 years earlier and an 87% response rate from 180 women who had the procedure 5 years earlier. Similar effects of NPV were seen on treatment outcome and need for reintervention. The overall reintervention rate was 43% at 3 years and 60% at 5 years. When stratifying according to NPV%, the reintervention rate in the 0%–25% NPV was 63% and 66% at 3 and 5 years, respectively; 40% and 63% at 3 and 5 years, respectively, in the 25%–50% NPV group; and 35% and 50% at 3 and 5 years, respectively, in the greater than 50% NPV group. This study also showed a relationship between increasing fibroid signal intensity and higher need for reintervention as a consequence of lower NPV that can be achieved in this fibroid type secondary to higher cell density.

It is important to note that the FDA initially limited the duration of the procedure to 3 hours for safety concerns. This time restriction significantly limited early treatment completion and success. Once procedure safety was documented and the time restrictions lifted, greater NPV could be achieved. Increased NPV along with increased operator experience will translate to improved outcomes with lower reintervention rates.

Risks

MRgFUS is tolerated well with low overall risk of side effects [19,21]. Most women reported mild pain during the procedure and mild-moderate pain that may last for up to 5 days. Minor complications described with this procedure include urinary tract infection, urinary retention, vaginal bleeding, transient buttock pain, and febrile morbidity. More serious complications are rare and may include fibroid expulsion, skin burns, and neuropathy. Thermal injury to surrounding viscera or nerves is an important but rare complication. Ultrasound energy is focused on the fibroid; however, lower levels are transmitted both forward and aft of the target. For example, sacral nerve palsy has been described occurring after sonication of a posterior fibroid that was near the pelvic bones [21]. Thus, it is imperative that the operator has a clean path to the target fibroid to minimize this risk. Ideal candidates are women who have a fibroid that leans up against the abdominal wall. The procedure cannot be done if the bladder, bowel, or nerves fall between the path of the ultrasound waves and the fibroid, or if the fibroid is directly apposed against any of these structures. Repositioning the patient can help to clear the field, but if critical structures cannot be moved and a clear path cannot be obtained, then the procedure cannot be performed.

Pregnancy Afterward

MRgFUS is currently approved for the treatment of women who do not desire future pregnancy. A study in 2010 by Rabinovici et al. detailed the outcomes of all pregnancies that had been reported up to that time after MRgFUS [23]. There were 54 pregnancies in 51 women. The outcomes were reassuring for typical pregnancy outcomes. Live births occurred in 41% of pregnancies, with a 28% spontaneous abortion rate, an 11% rate of elective pregnancy termination, and at the time this study was published, a 20% rate of ongoing pregnancies of greater than 20 weeks' gestational age. The vaginal delivery rate was 64%. Two patients had placental problems but had other risk factors for placental abnormalities.

Radiofrequency Ablation

The technique of RFA for the destruction of a lesion has long been utilized for various indications in medicine. RFA utilizes monopolar energy to induce coagulative necrosis. High-frequency alternating current (in the radiofrequency range, between 3 kHz and 300 GHz) is applied to a fibroid (or other tissue), causing tissue ions to oscillate and thus generating heat with subsequent protein denaturation and cell death. In 2002, Lee first described successfully treating fibroids with RFA, but it was not until 2012 that the first system designed for this indication was approved by the FDA (the Acessa System, Acessa Health) [24]. Because of the relative newness of this technique, data are limited compared to the previously discussed interventions.

Procedure Specifics

The RFA procedure is typically performed by a gynecologic surgeon. The patient is placed under general anesthesia in the operating room. A laparoscopic camera (5 or 10 mm) is commonly placed at the umbilicus through a standard port, and a laparoscopic ultrasound probe is placed through an additional port (10–12 mm), often suprapubic in location. The uterine fibroids are then mapped using both visual and laparoscopic guidance. The disposable, 3.4 mm, RFA handpiece is passed percutaneously (sans trocar) into the abdomen. Under both direct and sonographic guidance, the RFA handpiece is directed into a fibroid, the electrode array deployed, and the RFA cycle activated. The current is set at 460 kHz with a maximum output of 200 W. The generator displays tissue impedance, ablation time, and tissue temperature in real time. The goal is to reach a temperature of 100°C. The treatment time and generator settings are calculated based on an algorithm that factors the dimensions of the target myoma and deployment of needle array. For a large fibroid, multiple deployments within the same fibroid may be necessary. Once the necessary time at target temperature has been fulfilled, the electrode array is retracted. In an effort to protect the surrounding myometrium, a 0.5–1 cm safety barrier is necessary between the electrodes and the outside border of the fibroid.

Short-Term Outcomes

In 2013, Chudnoff et al. reported their outcomes from a multicenter, prospective clinical trial [25]. They included 137 patients with fibroids and at least a 6-month history of heavy menstrual bleeding. Patients were excluded if they had any of the following: MRI evidence of adenomyosis, type 0 submucosal fibroid, pedunculated subserosal fibroid, uterine size greater than 14 weeks, a single fibroid greater than 7 cm, and more than six total fibroids. The mean procedure length was 2.1 hours $\pm 1\%$, and 96% of patients were sent home the day of the procedure. Patients generally recovered well, and the median time to return to normal activities was 9 days (range 0–60 days), and the median missed days of work was 5 (range 0–29). At 12 months, 82% of patients reported a decrease in their menstrual blood loss, and 94% of patients reported satisfaction with the procedure. There was a 45% decrease in total mean myoma volume and a 38% reduction in menstrual blood loss.

Long-Term Outcomes and Reintervention

Because of the relative novelty of the Acessa RFA procedure, the longest follow-up data are 3 years postprocedure and were a continuation of the previously mentioned clinical trial [26]. Of the original 135 patients who underwent RFA, 104 were followed for the total 36 months. Using validated questionnaires, multiple subjective measures including symptom severity, health-related quality of life, and state of health, scores remained improved, suggesting persistent symptom relief over 3 years. The reintervention rate was 11%, or 14 of 135 participants. These interventions included 2 myomectomies, 11 hysterectomies, and 1 UAE. Half of the patients having repeat interventions were diagnosed with adenomyosis on pathology or imaging that had not been diagnosed at the time of study entry.

Risks

Similar to MRgFUS, RFA is a fibroid-specific therapy, so there is no risk of ovarian failure as can be seen with UAE. The procedure is safe with an overall low risk of complications. Device-related adverse events described in the original study included pelvic abscess requiring treatment with hospitalization, antibiotics, and drainage; a 2 cm sigmoid laceration from the ultrasound probe primarily repaired; vaginal bleeding; severe lower abdominal pain treated with NSAIDs; and mild superficial serosal burn that did not require intervention.

Pregnancy Afterward

RFA clinical trials have historically excluded women who desire future childbearing. Therefore, only case series of posttreatment pregnancies exist [27]. Twenty cases have been reported. There was one spontaneous abortion and seven elective terminations for undesired pregnancy. The remaining 12 pregnancies all went on to deliver at term, 75% by cesarean section and 25% by vaginal delivery. No uterine anomalies were reported. There was one delayed postpartum hemorrhage with expulsion of a degenerated fibroid. In this last case, a 4.7 cm transmural fibroid had been previously ablated. The patient required a blood transfusion and no further interventions.

Conclusion

UAE, MRgFUS, and RFA are associated with excellent clinical outcomes in the appropriately selected patient. It is of utmost importance to consider the patient's complaints and fibroid burden when selecting an intervention and counseling her about anticipated outcomes. Concurrent pathology, such as adenomyosis, endometriosis, and/or ovarian cysts, may also influence a patient's response to an intervention. There are few absolute restrictions to the size and number of fibroids that can be treated with each of these procedures, though increasing size of the uterus and/or fibroids predicts failure. Type 0 or type 1 submucosal fibroids as well as pedunculated subserosal fibroids are poor candidates for any of these procedures because of the risk of necrosis with expulsion. Favorable pregnancy outcomes have been described after each procedure; however, well-designed studies to examine pregnancy outcomes are lacking. Further, the exact effect of necrosis (coagulative or ischemic) on the uterus and surrounding myometrium and the effect of the degenerated fibroid(s) on uterine implantation, placentation, or contractility remain unknown.

REFERENCES

1. Das R, Champaneria R, Daniels JP, and Belli AM. Comparison of embolic agents used in uterine artery embolization: A systematic review and meta-analysis. *Cardiovasc Intervent Radiol*. 2014;37:1179–90.
2. Pron G, Cohen M, Soucie J, Garvin G, Vanderburgh L, Bell S, for the Ontario Uterine Fibroid Embolization Collaborative Group. The Ontario uterine fibroid embolization trial. Part 1. Baseline patient characteristics, fibroid burden and impact on life. *Fertil Steril*. 2003:79(1):112–9.
3. Pron G, Bennett J, Common A, Wall J, Asch M, Sniderman K, for the Ontario Uterine Fibroid Embolization Collaborative Group. The Ontario uterine fibroid embolization trial. Part 2. Uterine fibroid reduction and symptom relief after uterine artery embolization for fibroids. *Fertil Steril*. 2003:79(1):120–7.
4. Gupta JK, Sinha AS, Lumsden MA, and Hickey M. Uterine artery embolization for symptomatic uterine fibroids. *Cochrane Database Syst Rev*. 2014;(12):CD005073.
5. De Bruijn AM, Ankum WM, Reekers JA et al. Uterine artery embolization vs hysterectomy in the treatment of symptomatic uterine fibroids: 10-year outcomes from the randomized EMMY trial. *AJOG*. 2016;215:745.e1–12.
6. Hehenkamp WJ, Volkers NA, Birnie E, Reekers JA, and Ankum WM. Symptomatic uterine fibroids: Treatment with uterine artery embolization or hysterectomy. Results from the randomized clinical embolization versus hysterectomy (EMMY) trial. *Radiology*. 2008;246:823–32.
7. Spies JB, Ascher SA, Roth AR, Kim J, Levy EB, and Gomez-Jorge J. Uterine artery embolization for leiomyomata. *Obstet Gynecol*. 2001;98:29–34.
8. Walker WJ and Pelage JP. Uterine artery embolisation for symptomatic fibroids: Clinical results in 400 women with imaging follow up. *BJOG*. 2002;109:1262–72.
9. Van der Kooij SM, Bipat S, Hehendamp WJ, Ankum WM, and Reekers JA. Uterine artery embolization versus surgery in the treatment of symptomatic fibroids: A systematic review and metaanalysis. *Am J Obstet Gynecol*. 2011;205:317e1–18.
10. Spies JB, Myers ER, Worthington-Kirsch R, Mulgund J, Goodwin S, Mauro M; FIBROID Registry Investigators. The FIBROID registry: Symptom and quality of life status 1 year after therapy. *Obstet Gynecol*. 2005;106(6):1309–18.
11. Marret H, Cottier JP, Alonso AM, Giraudeau B, Body G, and Herbreteau D. Predictive factors for fibroid recurrence after uterine artery embolisation. *BJOG*. 2005;112:461–5.
12. Worthington-Kirsch R, Spies JB, Myers ER et al.; FIBROID Investigators. The fibroid registry for outcomes data (FIBROID) for uterine embolization: Short-term outcomes. *Obstet Gynecol*. 2005;106:52–9.
13. Vashisht A, Studd J, Carey A, and Burn P. Fatal septicaemia after fibroid embolization. *Lancet*. 1999;354:307–8.
14. Brown KT. Fatal pulmonary complications after arterial embolization with 40–120- micro m tris-acryl gelatin microspheres. *J Vasc Interv Radiol*. 2004;15:197–200.
15. Czeyda-Pommersheim F, Magee ST, Cooper C, Hahn WY, and Spies JB. Venous thromboembolism after uterine fibroid embolization. *Cardiovasc Intervent Radiol*. 2006;29:1136–40.
16. Homer H and Saridogan E. Uterine artery embolization for fibroids is associated with an increased risk of miscarriage. *Fertil Steril*. 2010;94(1):324–30.
17. Funaki K, Fukunishi H, and Sawada K. Clinical outcomes of magnetic resonance guided focused ultrasound surgery for uterine myomas: 24-month followup. *Ultrasound Obstet Gynecol*. 2009;34:584–9.
18. Jacoby VL, Kohi MP, Poder L et al. PROMISe trial: A pilot, randomized placebo-controlled trial of magnetic resonance guided focused ultrasound for uterine fibroids. *Gynecol Menopause*. 2016;105(3):773–80.
19. Stewart EA, Rabinovici J, Tempany CMC et al. Clinical outcomes of focused ultrasound surgery for the treatment of uterine fibroids. *Fertil Steril*. 2006;85(1):22–9.
20. Smart OC, Hindley JT, Regan L, and Gedroyc WG. Gonadotropin releasing hormone and magnetic resonance guided ultrasound surgery for uterine leiomyomata. *Obstet Gynecol*. 2006;108(1):49–54.

21. Quinn SD, Vedelago J, Geroyc W, and Regan L. Safety and five year re-intervention following magnetic resonance guided focused ultrasound (MRgFUS) for uterine fibroids. *Eur J Obstet Gynecol Reprod Biol.* 2014;182:247–51.

22. Stewart EA, Gostout B, Rabinovici J, Kim HS, Regan L, and Tempany CMC. Sustained relief of leiomyoma symptoms by using focused ultrasound surgery. *Obstet Gynecol.* 2007;110(2):279–87.

23. Rabinovici J, David M, Fukunishi H, Morita Y, Gostout B, Stewart EA; MRgFUS Study Group. Pregnancy outcome after magnetic resonance guided focused ultrasound surgery (MRgFUS) for conservative treatment of uterine fibroids. *Fertil Steril.* 2010;93:199–209.

24. Lee BB. Radiofrequency ablation of uterine leiomyomata: A new minimally invasive hysterectomy alternative. *Obstet Gynecol.* 2002;99(4s):9s.

25. Chudnoff SG, Berman JM, Levine DJ, Harris M, Guido RS, and Banks E. Outpatient procedure for the treatment and relief of symptomatic uterine myomas. *Obstec Gynecol.* 2013;121(5):1075–82.

26. Berman JM, Guido RS, Garza-Leal JG, Pemueller RR, Whaley FS, and Chudnoff SG. Three-year outcome of the halt trial; a prospective analysis of radiofrequency volumetric thermal ablation of myomas. *J Min Inv Gynecol.* 2014;21(5):767–74.

27. Keltz J, Levie M, and Chudnoff S. Pregnancy outcomes after direct uterine myoma thermal ablation: Review of the literature. *JMIG.* 2017;24(4):538–45.

10

Hysteroscopic Myomectomy

Anja Frost and Mostafa A. Borahay

CONTENTS

Evolution of Hysteroscopic Myomectomy

The procedure of hysteroscopic resection of fibroids was first described in 1976 by Neuwirth and Amin using a urologic resectoscope as a surgical method to avoid abdominal surgery. With multiple modifications of equipment and improvements in technique, resection of submucosal fibroids using hysteroscopy has become the first-line surgical option and the gold standard for many submucosal fibroids with or without intramural components (International Federation of Gynecology and Obstetrics [FIGO] type 0-2; see Figure 2.2 in Chapter 2) [1,2]. There are many benefits to this surgical approach, including avoidance of laparotomy (and conventional or robotic-assisted laparoscopy), which decreases the chance for several complications, a significantly shortened postoperative recovery, and possible performance in an ambulatory setting. Additionally, with the avoidance of hysterotomy, the need for future cesarean section is significantly reduced, which improves pregnancy outcomes in childbearing women.

Significance of Submucosal Fibroids

The most significant symptom of submucosal fibroids is abnormal uterine bleeding, most commonly described as heavy or prolonged menstrual bleeding [3]. The prevalence of submucosal fibroids in women with abnormal uterine bleeding was found to be 23.4%, with the majority of these being premenopausal women [4]. Multiple studies have shown rates of menstrual symptoms improvement of 62%–90%, defined as a "surgery-free" interval at 5 years [5,6].

Submucosal fibroids can play a significant role regarding both infertility and early pregnancy loss. Uterine fibroids have been detected in 5%–10% of women with infertility; in 1%–2.4% of women with infertility, uterine fibroids have been the only abnormality noted on comprehensive workup [7]. Higher spontaneous abortion rates have been noted among women with submucosal myomas, and this difference seems to disappear following hysteroscopic myomectomy [8]. Mechanisms of myomas causing infertility or early pregnancy loss are still under investigation, but it is thought that the endometrium overlying submucosal myomas displays glandular atrophy, which can prohibit implantation and growth of the developing embryo [9].

Preoperative Imaging

Multiple preoperative modalities can be used to map intracavitary fibroids, including transvaginal ultrasound (TVUS), saline infusion sonography (SIS), magnetic resonance imaging (MRI), and office hysteroscopy. TVUS is generally the first-line modality given its widespread availability and relative low cost; however, it is not only operator dependent but most accurate when assessing small uteri with four or less fibroids [10]. Clinicians should view the images themselves preoperatively, as the appropriateness and approach to surgical planning are highly dependent on quality and proper interpretation of imaging, which can be variable with ultrasound imaging. Although TVUS cannot assess the degree of intracavitary extension of the fibroid, it can show the thickness of the outer myometrial layer of the fibroid as well as the presence of any other possible associated pathology.

SIS is able to delineate submucosal fibroids and evaluate their relation to the endometrial cavity. MRI has been shown to have 100% sensitivity and 91% specificity in detecting submucosal fibroids, outperforming TVUS, SIS, and even hysteroscopy, especially with regard to reproducibility, although it is a far more expensive approach and is not always available [11]. Doppler and three-dimensional (3D) ultrasound are often helpful to differentiate between adenomyosis and leiomyomas as well as demarcate vascular patterns surrounding fibroids [12]. Therapeutic approaches for adenomyosis versus leiomyomas are very different; therefore, this distinction is often crucial prior to myomectomy.

Patient Selection

The classification of submucosal fibroids was first described by Wamsteker et al. in 1993 and is now universally used [13]. Type 0 includes pedunculated fibroids completely within the cavity, type 1 with less than 50% myometrial extension, and type 2 with greater than 50% myometrial extension [2]. Generally, type 0 or 1 myomas are considered resectable with a single hysteroscopic operation in most instances, while type 2 fibroids can require a larger number of repeat or two-staged procedures [13]. See further Chapter 1.

Patients with symptomatic submucosal fibroids including, but not limited to, heavy or abnormal bleeding, infertility (generally type 0 or 1), or recurrent pregnancy loss, are potential candidates for myomectomy [3]. Patients are selected based on fibroid number, type, size, and location; patient parity; and other comorbidities. Knowledge of these variables allows appropriate patient counseling regarding success of complete resection, risk of needing additional surgery for complete removal, recurrence rate, as well as surgical planning for technique of removal.

Proper patient selection is required to ensure safety and feasibility of the procedure, and historically the degree of intramural involvement and size of fibroid have been noted to be the most important factors in predicting a normal postoperative cavity. It is critical to gain accurate information on the thickness of the myometrium between the intramural portion of the submucosal fibroid and the uterine serosa. Data have shown that if the thickness is less than 5 mm that the risk of uterine perforation outweighs the benefit of a hysteroscopic approach, and 5–10 mm is recommended [14].

Generally, intracavitary fibroids less than 4 cm have been shown to have safe and effective outcomes with hysteroscopic myomectomy; however, a two-step resection is possible with 4–6 cm intracavitary fibroids. With fibroids over 6 cm, data have shown increased rates of secondary procedures, longer recovery time, and incomplete resection or resolution of symptoms [15]. Certain studies have shown that a fibroid diameter of less than 2.6 cm and greater than 65% extension into the cavity can predict a high probability of complete resection with a single hysteroscopic myomectomy [2]. The projected risk of additional surgical intervention within 5 years for two or less submucosal fibroids with a normal uterine size is approximately 10%, while the risk increases significantly with three or more submucosal fibroids and an enlarged uterus with a risk of 35% [3]. Additionally, the location of the fibroid is critical, as fibroids located close to the cornua may result in ablation or occlusion of the tubal ostia following hysteroscopic removal [16].

Overall, it is important to consider myoma type, significance of the patient's symptoms, risk of incomplete excision, and the patient's tolerance for and acceptance of additional procedures.

Preoperative Considerations (Cervical Ripening, Antibiotics, Venous Thromboembolism Prophylaxis)

Multiple interventions have been studied to facilitate cervical ripening with generally conflicting results. The goal of cervical ripening is to avoid complications, such as creations of a false passage, cervical tears, and uterine perforation; as well as to facilitate greater ease of procedure, likely to be considered more in operative versus diagnostic hysteroscopy. The use of misoprostol (vaginal, oral, or sublingual) in some studies has shown to be more effective in decreasing the need for cervical dilation than placebo in premenopausal but not in postmenopausal women. In addition, some studies showed misoprostol to decrease complications (as cervical laceration and false tracks), while others did not. Finally, misoprostol has side effects such as cramps, bleeding, nausea, and diarrhea [17–19]. One must, of course, take into account the parity of the patient, as cervical ripening for a diagnostic hysteroscopy in a multiparous woman is likely to be superfluous.

Pretreatment with a gonadotropin-releasing hormone (GnRH) agonist has been shown to be beneficial for improving anemia due to an induced state of amenorrhea, reduction of endometrial thickness and vascularization of fibroids, and allowance of timing of surgery not only limited to the early proliferative phase. Most studies have shown the greatest benefit of GnRH agonist treatment in larger fibroids (greater than 3–4 cm) with concurrent anemia (see further Chapter 6). The most useful effects of GnRH agonists are reduced operating time and decreased hysteroscopic fluid resorption; however, no difference was noted in complete resection or need for repeat operation [20]. That being said, it is important to consider the high costs, side effects, and possible increased risk of uterine perforation due to decreased myometrial thickness. Details regarding dosing and administration timing are discussed in Chapters 6 and 11. Ulipristal acetate has shown preoperative reduction in size of fibroids and decreased vaginal bleeding. One can consider usage of 5 or 10 mg daily dosing prior to operation (up to 13 weeks) [21]. Additional or alternative use of laminaria or adjunct estrogen has yielded inconsistent results [22,23]. In summary, there are not yet consistent guidelines for cervical preparation prior to hysteroscopy and should be determined on a case-by-case basis based on age, parity, in-office exam, and imaging results.

Regarding preoperative prophylaxis, no antibiotic prophylaxis is recommended for hysteroscopic myomectomy. Venous thromboembolic prophylaxis should follow a risk-based approach, although it is rarely necessary.

Consents

Topics to discuss with patients include intraoperative expectations as well as long-term risks. It is important to discuss risks of bleeding and infection, although the risk of both should be minimal with hysteroscopic myomectomy. The risk of uterine perforation and possible laparoscopy must be discussed and should be added to consent forms. Regarding long-term postoperative measures, it is important to counsel patients that there is both a risk of recurrence (discussed more later) as well as a risk of incomplete resolution of symptoms based on either the size and/or myometrial extension of their fibroids, or the possibility of additional/alternative pathologies playing a role in their abnormal uterine bleeding. If myomectomy is being performed for fertility reasons, it is important to counsel patients that it is rare for submucosal fibroids to be the sole cause of infertility and that this procedure may not return the patients to baseline fertility levels or ensure successful subsequent *in vitro* fertilization.

Surgical Steps, Intraoperative Considerations, and Complication Prevention

The patient should be in low dorsal lithotomy position in support stirrups after anesthesia induction, consisting of either sedation or general anesthesia. A bimanual exam should be performed to assess size and flexion of the uterus in order to minimize uterine perforation.

Cervical injection of vasopressin can be considered before the start of the case, which can reduce intravasation of fluid, reduce intraoperative blood loss, and improve visualization, although it has not been shown to reduce operation duration [24]. Paracervical/intracervical blockade has also been studied and can be considered with injection of local anesthetic (i.e., 1% lidocaine) prior to initiation of cervical dilation.

Close attention should be paid to avoiding uterine perforation, which can happen at any time during the procedure from uterine sounding, cervical dilation, hysteroscope insertion, and/or during fibroid resection. Perforation occurring at the time of cervical dilation is most commonly due to cervical stenosis, a severely retro- or anteverted uterus, or in nulliparous/menopausal women. If uterine perforation is recognized, it is important to identify which steps of the hysteroscopy have been completed thus far; regardless, the procedure should be terminated. If only a mechanical perforation without suspicion of bowel damage, patients can be placed in extended observation for a few additional hours and discharged home. If perforation is secondary to an activated electrode or sharp instrument, one should assume the possibility of bowel injury, and diagnostic laparoscopy should be performed immediately. If perforation is noted, the perforation should be sutured in patients of reproductive age even if hemostatic due to the risk of uterine rupture during pregnancy [25].

Once all equipment has been set up and hysteroscopy can commence, a distending media is used (described in more detail later). The decision for fluid distention (both fluid type and distending pressure) should be based on the procedure planned, and it is critical to be familiar with possible complications and acceptable fluid deficits. Fluid deficit is the difference between the total amount of solution instilled into the uterus and the amount of fluid recovered from the hysteroscope outlet channel and the plastic draping pouch used to funnel escaping fluid through the cervix through a tube into a calibrated bottle. Many fluid management systems can measure both instilled and recovered fluid and give the fluid deficit on the machine control panel. The surgeon should continue to communicate with operating room staff regarding fluid deficit over time in order to plan the timing of the remainder of the surgery, and if all specimens can be removed safely in line with fluid deficit restrictions.

Three types of distending media are available: carbon dioxide gas, hypotonic nonconductive fluid (glycine, sorbitol, mannitol), and isotonic conductive fluids (normal saline). Carbon dioxide is only available for diagnostic use and because it has a risk of gas embolization, it is not discussed further with regard to operative hysteroscopic surgery in this chapter. Hypotonic fluids like those described earlier are used with monopolar energy and can have significant complications, such as volume overload, water intoxication, pulmonary edema, severe hyponatremia, and cerebral edema. Isotonic fluids used with bipolar energy are generally better tolerated with the most common complication being fluid overload, generally easily treatable with diuretics. Regardless of the fluid medium, steps should be taken to minimize fluid intravasation, especially in cases with increased risk with larger intracavitary component. Complications can be avoided with strict tracking of fluid deficit and using the minimum fluid pressure for visualization, which is generally between 60 and 80 mm Hg, dependent on the patient's mean arterial pressure (MAP) [26]. The American Association of Gynecologic Laparoscopists recommends a maximum fluid deficit of 750 mL for elderly patients or those with cardiac comorbidities and 1000 and 2500 mL for younger, healthy patients with hypotonic and isotonic solutions, respectively [27].

Diagnostic hysteroscopy, most commonly with a rigid 5 mm hysteroscope, is recommended prior to initiation of operative hysteroscopy to confirm imaging findings and to determine the surgical plan. The most common angles for visualization are 12° and 30°. An outer sheath is generally necessary to allow for inflow and outflow channels for fluid distention and generation of a lavage system for the uterine cavity for improved visualization. Cervical dilation is generally not necessary in most patients prior to diagnostic hysteroscopy, although special consideration for nulliparous or menopause women should be made which may require dilation.

Instruments, Devices, and Special Techniques

Operative hysteroscopes, also described as resectoscopes, generally range from 6 mm to 10 mm in diameter and contain a working element using electrosurgical loops, mechanical cold loops, or morcellator technology (Figure 10.1). There are several methods to resect submucosal fibroids hysteroscopically including monopolar resection, bipolar resection using loop resection, traditional mechanical methods

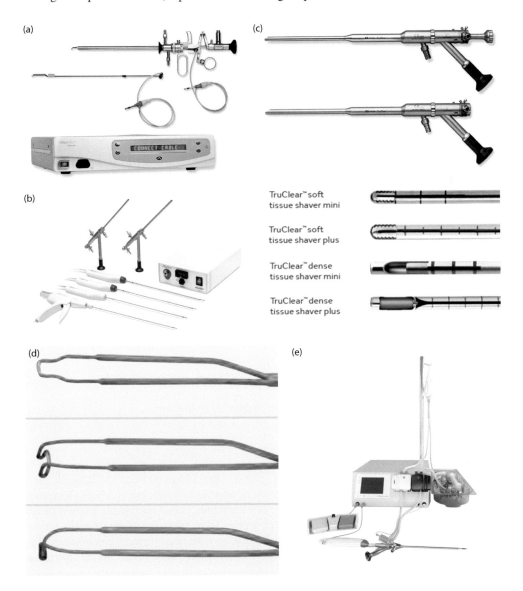

FIGURE 10.1 Hysteroscopic tissue removal devices. (a) Versapoint System. (From Gynecare Versapoint Bipolar Electrosurgery System; Helpful Hints from Ethicon at https://www.ethicon.com/na/system/files/2018-05/027687-150113_VP_HelpfulHints_5_CR.pdf, with permission.) (b) MyoSure System. (From MyoSure Tissue Removal Procedure Physician Brochure from Hologic at https://gynsurgicalsolutions.com/product/myosure-tissue-removal/, with permission.) (c) TruClear System. (From TruClear Hysteroscopic Tissue Removal System brochure from Medtronic at https://www.medtronic.com/content/dam/covidien/library/us/en/product/gynecology-products/truclear-system-comprehensive-brochure.pdf, with permission.) (d) Mazzon cold loops. (From Karl Storz; at https://www.karlstorz.com/cps/rde/xbcr/karlstorz_assets/ASSETS/3343847.pdf, with permission.) (e) Symphion System. (From Symphion Tissue Removal System from Boston Scientific at http://www.bostonscientific.com/content/gwc/en-US/products/uterine-tissue-removal-systems/symphion-system.html, with permission.)

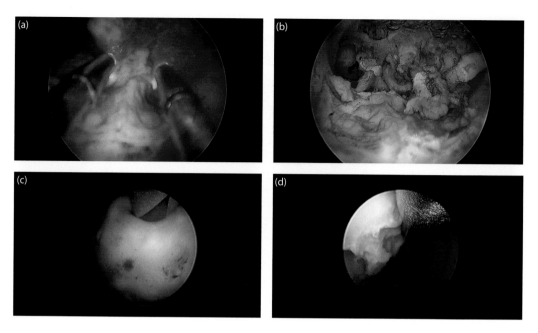

FIGURE 10.2 (a) Hysteroscopic view of submucosal leiomyoma resection using Versapoint bipolar resectoscope. (b) Hysteroscopic view of leiomyoma fragments following myomectomy using Versapoint. (c) Hysteroscopic view of submucosal leiomyoma resection using MyoSure device. (d) Hysteroscopic view of submucosal leiomyoma resection using MyoSure device.

VIDEO 10.1   Segment of submucosal leiomyoma resection using Versapoint bipolar resectoscope.

URL: https://youtu.be/xEkkwGQYp8Q

VIDEO 10.2   Segment of submucosal leiomyoma resection using MyoSure device.

URL: https://youtu.be/cAaZvpu5Fmk

---

with scissors, or newer hysteroscopic morcellation. Figure 10.2 and Videos 10.1 and 10.2 illustrate some of the views and techniques of hysteroscopic myomectomy. Bipolar instruments, in which both electrodes are introduced into the thermal loop, are generally safer as current only passes through the tissue with which the loop comes into contact, minimizing the danger derived from random passage from the corporeal structures. While other methods exist, such as vaporization with laser therapy, electrosurgical loop resection is the most commonly performed. When dealing with small submucosal fibroids, particularly in patients with infertility, it might be ideal to avoid electrosurgery in order to decrease adhesion rate.

There are multiple devices (Figure 10.1) in use for myomectomy, including traditional electrocautery resectoscopes (most common is Versapoint by Ethicon, Mazzon cold loops by Karl Storz, as well as intrauterine morcellators [IUMs]). IUM systems, including Truclear by Smith & Nephews, MyoSure by Hologic, and Symphion by Boston Scientific, are all-in-one, self-contained recirculating fluid systems, direct internal pressure monitors, and bladeless bipolar resection devices. IUM systems have a sheathed cutting blade without electrosurgical energy and vacuum suction for simultaneous tissue resection and removal. This removes the time-consuming nature of repeat manual extraction of shaved fragments for improved visualization. Benefits of these devices include improved complete resection, low complication rates (less than 1%), faster removal, and reduced mean operating time. One must take caution with fibroids greater than 4 cm, as often there is a lower complete resection rate with morcellation devices and more need for conversion to electrosurgical technique, especially with a significant intramural component [28,29].

If pedunculated submucosal fibroids are noted (type 0), the base of the pedicle can generally be transected easily with the electrosurgical loop and is generally performed using a slicing technique of the cutting loop until normal myometrial fibers can be noted (more vascular and pink-appearing layer of tissue). The fibroid can then be extracted either with the loop or sometimes blindly with a curette or grasper. With type 1 or 2 fibroids, the procedure can become somewhat more complex, which may require multiple rounds of resection of the fibroid from the intracavitary layer up toward the myometrium. The Mazzon technique, with a described up to 88% success rate in one-step surgical removal of type 1 and 2 fibroids, uses cold loop to minimize both thermal damage to healthy myometrium as well as decrease synechiae formation. Mechanical enucleation of intramural components over slicing not only respects the anatomy and integrity of the myometrium but also avoids significant risks such as thermal perforation [30].

Another technique has been described by Zayed et al. for successful one-stage procedures for fibroids with intramural components. This involves using a U-shaped cutting loop to slice down to the level of the endometrial surface, then inserting the resectoscope loop into the cleavage plane between the myoma and myometrium to bring the intramural component into the uterine cavity. Saline infusion would then be discontinued and restarted multiple times to induce rapid intrauterine pressure changes and stimulate contractions as well as act as a component of bimanual massage. This technique has been successful with 95% success in removal for type II fibroids less than 6 cm [31].

Office Myomectomy

Office hysteroscopy is generally feasible and safe for both diagnosis and occasionally treatment of small intrauterine pathologies, which is often referred to as the "see and treat" approach. Office hysteroscopy can be considered with less than 5 mm hysteroscopes to minimize the risk of cervical dilation, need for anesthesia, and costs. The other benefits include immediate resumption of normal activities postprocedure, when nonsteroidal anti-inflammatory drugs alone are used, and although pain is the primary reason for aborting in-office procedures, the use of opioid medications or anxiolytics has not shown any added benefit. Outpatient office-based resection of types 0-1 fibroids less than 1.5 cm, polyps resected with direct visualization, and adhesiolysis with hysteroscopic scissors have been found to be safe and well-tolerated procedures. The most common complications from in-office hysteroscopy include vasovagal reaction, local anesthesia toxicity, uterine perforation, uterine hemorrhage, and false passages. It is recommended that both office and clinical staff undertake a safety self-assessment and practice simulated patient scenarios at regular intervals to be prepared for situations with procedural complications. If only a 5 mm hysteroscope or less is used, pelvic rest is not required. Setup and precautions of office hysteroscopic procedures should be adopted [32].

Postoperative Care

Postoperative care is generally straightforward, and patients should be discharged home the same day unless any of the complications mentioned earlier were to occur requiring extended observation or management (perforation, excessive fluid intravasation). There are no restrictions on return to normal activity following hysteroscopic myomectomy, and patients should be able to shower when they return home after surgery. Patients should be counseled that vaginal spotting can occur for up to 4 weeks after surgery, although strict precautions for heavy bleeding (changing two pads per hour for over 2 hours), fevers, foul-smelling discharge, or severe abdominal pain should prompt reevaluation prior to the postoperative visit.

Outcomes (Recurrence, Fertility, Adhesions)

Recurrence of symptoms and reoperation rates vary greatly based on age, presenting symptoms, number of fibroids removed, and types of fibroids removed. Data have shown that there is an approximate 30% 3-year cumulative recurrence rate with reoperation rates of approximately 5%–20% at 3–4 years [26,33].

After all other causes of infertility have been evaluated and addressed, fertility outcomes after hysteroscopic myomectomy are favorable with an increase in pregnancy rates, higher live birth rates, and less miscarriages [8]. It is recommended that women wait around 2–3 weeks following myomectomy to resume fertility attempts to ensure proper healing of the uterine cavity.

Adhesion rates after cold loop and energy resection are estimated at 4% and 30%, respectively. After monopolar and bipolar energy, adhesion rates are estimated at 35%–40% and 7.5%, respectively [34]. Certain studies have shown the benefit of application of auto-cross-linked hyaluronan (ACH), an antiadhesion agent; however, overall data are inconclusive, and therefore, there is currently no guideline or recommendation for the use of these agents [35,36]. Therefore, using special care to avoid trauma to healthy endometrium and myometrium, reducing the risk of electrosurgery when possible, and avoiding forced cervical manipulation are the best tactics at this time. Early second-look hysteroscopy is not recommended. The possibility of uterine rupture is addressed more often in laparoscopic myomectomy; however, if hysteroscopic myomectomy invades the myometrium or a perforation during entry or surgery occurs, this should be discussed with the patient and clearly documented in the medical records.

Conclusion

Hysteroscopic myomectomy is a significant advancement in the field of hysteroscopic surgery and continues to evolve with new devices and techniques. Not only is this a quick, cost-effective procedure, but excellent results have been noted both with regard to irregular bleeding and improvement in fertility. Success of the procedure must always be individualized to patient risk factors; number, type, size, and location of fibroids; and goal of the procedure.

REFERENCES

1. Christian SS and Schlaff WD. Hysteroscopic myomectomy. In: Azziz R and Murphy AA (eds) *Practical Manual of Operative Laparoscopy and Hysteroscopy*. New York, NY: Springer; 1997.
2. Keltz MD, Greene AD, Morrissey MB, Vega M, and Moshier E. Sono-hysterographic predictors of successful hysteroscopic myomectomies. *JSLS*. 2015;19(01):00105.
3. American Association of Gynecologic Laparoscopists (AAGL): Advancing Minimally Invasive Gynecology Worldwide. AAGL practice report: Practice guidelines for the diagnosis and management of submucous leiomyomas. *J Minim Invasive Gynecol*. 2012;19(02):152–71.
4. van Dongen H, de Kroon CD, Jacobi CE, Trimbos JB, and Jansen FW. Diagnostic hysteroscopy in abnormal uterine bleeding: A systematic review and meta-analysis. *BJOG*. 2007;114:664–75.
5. Emanuel MH, Wamsteker K, Hart AA, Metz G, and Lammes FB. Long-term results of hysteroscopic myomectomy for abnormal uterine bleeding. *Obstet Gynecol*. 1999;93:743–8.
6. Fernandez H, Sefrioui O, Virelizier C, Gervaise A, Gomel V, and Frydman R. Hysteroscopic resection of submucosal myomas in patients with infertility. *Hum Reprod*. 2001;16:1489–92.
7. Buttram VC Jr and Reiter RC. Uterine leiomyomata: Etiology, symptomatology, and management. *Fertil Steril*. 1981;36:433–45.
8. Pritts EA, Parker WH, and Olive DL. Fibroids and infertility: An updated systematic review of the evidence. *Fertil Steril*. 2009;91:1215–23.
9. Maguire M, and Segars JH. Benign uterine disease: Leiomyomata and benign polyps. In: Aplin JD, Fazleabas AT, Glasser SR, and Giudice LC (eds). *The Endometrium: Molecular, Cellular and Clinical Perspectives*. 2nd ed. London: Informa Health Care; 2008.
10. Falcone T and Parker WH. Surgical management of leiomyomas for fertility or uterine preservation. *Obstet Gynecol*. 2013;121:856–68.

11. Closon F and Tulandi T. Future research and developments in hysteroscopy. *Best Pract Res Clin Obstet Gynaecol*. 2015;29:994–1000.

12. Nieuwhenhuis LL, Betjes HE, Hehenkamp WJ et al. The use of 3D power Doppler ultrasound in the quantification of blood vessels in uterine fibroids: Feasibility and reproducibility. *J Clin Ultrasound*. 2013;43:171–8.

13. Wamsteker K, Emanuel MH, and de Kruif JH. Transcervical hysteroscopic resection of submucous fibroids for abnormal uterine bleeding: Results regarding the degree of intramural extension, *Obstet Gynecol*. 1993;82:736–40.

14. Lewis EI and Gargiulo AR. The role of hysteroscopic and robot-assisted laparoscopic myomectomy in the setting of infertility. *Clin Obstet Gynecol*. 2016;59(1):53–65.

15. Di Spiezio Sardo A, Mazzon I, Bramante S et al. Hysteroscopic myomectomy: A comprehensive review of surgical techniques. *Hum Reprod Update*. 2008;14(2):101–19.

16. Pakrashi T. New hysteroscopic techniques for submucosal uterine fibroid. *Curr Opin Obstet Gynecol*. 2013;26:308–13.

17. Gkrozou F, Koliopoulos G, Vrekoussis T et al. A systematic review and meta-analysis of randomized studies comparing misoprostol versus placebo for cervical ripening prior to hysteroscopy. *Eur J Obstet Gynecol Reprod Biol*. 2011;158(1):17–23.

18. Selk A and Kroft J. Misoprostol in operative hysteroscopy: A systematic review and meta-analysis. *Obstet Gynecol*. 2011;118(4):941–9.

19. Polyzos NP, Zavos A, Valachis A et al. Misoprostol prior to hysteroscopy in premenopausal and post-menopausal women. A systematic review and meta-analysis. *Hum Reprod Update*. 2012;18(4):393–404.

20. Kamath MS, Kalampokas EE, and Kalampokas TE. Use of GnRH analogues pre-operatively for hysteroscopic resection of submucous fibroids: A systematic review and meta-analysis. *Eur J Obstet Gynecol Reprod Biol*. 2014;177:11–8.

21. Donnez J, Tatarchuk TF, Bouchard P et al.; PEARL I Study Group. Ulipristal acetate versus placebo for fibroid treatment before surgery. *N Engl J Med*. 2012;366(05):409–20.

22. Darwish AM, Ahmad AM, and Mohammad AM. Cervical priming prior to operative hysteroscopy: A randomized comparison of laminaria versus misoprostol. *Hum Reprod*. 2004;19(10):2391–4.

23. Oppegaard KS, Lieng M, Berg A, Istre O, Qvigstad E, and Nesheim BI. A combination of misoprostol and estradiol for preoperative cervical ripening in postmenopausal women: A randomised controlled trial. *BJOG*. 2010;117(1):53–61.

24. Wong ASW, Cheung CW, Yeung SW et al. Transcervical intralesional vasopressin injection compared with placebo in hysteroscopic myomectomy: A randomized controlled trial. *Obstet Gynecol*. 2014;124(5):897–903.

25. Indman PD. Hysteroscopic treatment of submucous fibroids. *Clin Obstet Gynecol*. 2006;49:811–20.

26. Emanuel MH. Hysteroscopy and the treatment of uterine fibroids. *Best Pract Res Clin Obstet Gynaecol*. 2015;29(7):920–9.

27. Munro MG, Storz K, Abbott JA et al.; AAGL Advancing Minimally Invasive Gynecology Worldwide. AAGL practice report: Practice guidelines for the management of hysteroscopic distending media: Replaces hysteroscopic fluid monitoring guidelines. *J Am Assoc Gynecol Laparosc*. 2000;7:167–8. *J Minim Invasive Gynecol*. 2013;20(02):137–48.

28. Haber K, Hawkins E, Levie M, and Chudnoff S. Hysteroscopic morcellation: Review of the manufacturer and user facility device experience (MAUDE) database. *J Minim Invasive Gynecol*. 2015;22(01):110–4.

29. Hamerlynck TW, Dietz V, and Schoot BC. Clinical implementation of the hysteroscopic morcellator for removal of intrauterine myomas and polyps. A retrospective descriptive study. *Gynecol Surg*. 2011;8(02):193–6.

30. Mazzon I, Favilli A, Grasso M, Horvath S, Di Renzo GC, and Gerli S. Is cold loop hysteroscopic myomectomy a safe and effective technique for the treatment of submucous myomas with intramural development? A series of 1434 surgical procedures. *J Minim Invasive Gynecol*. 2015;22(5):792–8.

31. Zayed M, Fouda UM, Zayed SM, Elsetohy KA, and Hashem AT. Hysteroscopic myomectomy of large submucous myomas in a 1-step procedure using multiple slicing sessions technique. *J Minim Invasive Gynecol*. 2015;22(07):1196–202.

32. Salazar CA and Isaacson KB. Office operating hysteroscopy: An update. *J Minim Invasive Gynecol*. 2018;25(2):199–208.

33. Vercellini P, Zàina B, Yaylayan L, Pisacreta A, De Giorgi O, and Crosignani PG. Hysteroscopic myomectomy: Long-term effects on menstrual pattern and fertility. *Obstet Gynecol.* 1999;94(3):341–7.
34. Capmas P, Levaillant JM, and Fernandez H. Review surgical techniques and outcome in the management of submucous fibroids. *Curr Opin Obstet Gynecol.* 2013;25(4):332–8.
35. Mais V, Cirronis MG, Peiretti M, Ferrucci G, Cossu E, and Melis GB. Efficacy of auto-crosslinked hyaluronan gel for adhesion prevention in laparoscopy and hysteroscopy: A systematic review and meta-analysis of randomized controlled trials. *Eur J Obstet Gynecol Reprod Biol.* 2012;160(1):1–5.
36. Bosteels J, Weyers S, Mol BW, and D'Hooghe T. Anti-adhesion barrier gels following operative hysteroscopy for treating female infertility: A systematic review and meta-analysis. *Gynecol Surg.* 2014;11:113–27.

11

Laparoscopic and Robotic-Assisted Myomectomy

Harold Wu, Anja Frost, and Mostafa A. Borahay

CONTENTS

Patient Evaluation and Selection

Laparoscopic myomectomy (LM), with or without robotic assistance, is the minimally invasive surgical approach of choice for the fertility-sparing management of most symptomatic intramural and subserosal fibroids. Accurate evaluation of the fibroids is of paramount importance for proper preoperative and intraoperative surgical planning to ensure complete excision, especially given the lack of ability to directly palpate the fibroids during laparoscopy. Though pelvic ultrasonography is considered the gold standard for the diagnosis of fibroids, magnetic resonance imaging (MRI) is a useful tool for further surgical planning. MRI can reliably assess several characteristics of fibroids, including number, size, location, relationship to the intrauterine cavity, surrounding normal myometrium/serosal surface, involvement of or extension into surrounding pelvic structures, and vascularization patterns.

Criteria proposed for a laparoscopic (LSC) approach to myomectomy have been quite variable, and there are no standardized guidelines. Studies have suggested an increased risk of complications with multiple, large fibroids, and fibroids located in an intraligamental location [1]. Some surgeons have suggested avoiding a LSC approach with more than four fibroids or large fibroids (greater than 10–12 cm); others have recommended a uterus less than 16 weeks' size, less than five fibroids, and no single fibroid greater than 15 cm [2,3]. Furthermore, fibroids that involve the cervix, broad ligament, and uterine cornu may increase the risk of conversion to hysterectomy. An open approach may be preferred when adequate exposure to key anatomic structures is difficult or a need for significant uterine reconstruction is anticipated. Ultimately, surgeon experience and comfort with laparoscopic dissection should determine the number, size, and location of fibroids that can be adequately and safely resected while optimizing myometrial closure and tissue integrity.

Preoperative Management

Several management options are available preoperatively to address significant patient anemia from abnormal uterine bleeding, as well as decrease tumor size/burden to decrease intraoperative blood loss and facilitate surgical removal of the fibroids. Iron supplementation to correct anemia can be through oral or parenteral routes. Autologous transfusion or cell saver devices, in addition to cross-matched packed red blood cells, can be prepared for surgery if significant blood loss is expected.

The most extensively studied medication in this preoperative management setting is gonadotropin-releasing hormone agonist (GnRHa) therapy, which has been known to shrink fibroid volume by 35% within 8 weeks of therapy (in addition to induction of amenorrhea), with up to 70% reduction by 24 weeks [4,5]. Studies have noted a reduction in estimated blood loss (EBL, mean 60 cc), reduction in operative times (mean 25.8 minutes), and increase in postoperative hemoglobin (mean 1.15 g/dL) [6,7]. However, it is important to counsel patients regarding menopausal symptoms that may be poorly tolerated and limit treatment duration even despite estrogen add-back therapy. Furthermore, GnRHa therapy may also distort pseudocapsule planes, making fibroid enucleation and dissection more difficult. Other options for medical pretreatment include ulipristal acetate (UPA), of which 3 months of treatment has been shown to be noninferior to leuprolide acetate in managing heavy bleeding prior to surgery with less likelihood of hot flashes [8]. Cotreatment of letrozole and norethindrone acetate for 3 months has been shown to reduce operative time (mean 12.9 minutes) and EBL (189.4 cc) with better-defined surgical planes [9].

Uterine artery embolization (UAE), often performed by interventional radiologists, causes ischemic necrosis of fibroids (while normal myometrium vascularizes) via a minimally invasive angiographic approach. The procedure can reduce fibroid volumes up to 49% by 6 months [10]. Notably, aside from facilitating surgery for larger fibroids, studies have not found significantly decreased operative times or EBL [11]. It is important to counsel patients regarding the controversial nature of UAE with respect to future fertility. While some studies have shown no effects from UAE on fertility rates and perinatal/obstetrical outcomes, others showed greater rates of spontaneous abortions, abnormal placentation, and cesarean sections [10,12–16].

Consents and Outcomes

Several important points should be discussed with patients at the time of the consenting process. Intraoperative bleeding at the time of the myomectomy may be significant enough to warrant a blood transfusion. Uncontrolled hemorrhage or extensive disruption of the myometrium may necessitate a hysterectomy. The risk of conversion to an open procedure is generally quoted from 2% to 8% [17].

Despite adequate tumor removal at the time of surgery, fibroids can recur, especially in reproductive-age women remote from menopause. Indeed, one study found that age 30–40 years and more than one fibroid at the time of surgery were significantly associated with symptomatic recurrence [18]. Reported rates of recurrence and reoperation in LM are variable. While an older study cited the 5-year cumulative recurrence risk to be as high as approximately 50% with a 12% reoperation rate, newer studies have found it at approximately 15%–20% with a much lower 4% reoperation rate [18–20].

The disruption of healthy myometrium and uterine integrity during a myomectomy raises significant concern for possible uterine rupture during subsequent pregnancies and labor. Women planning to undergo a myomectomy for fertility-sparing reasons should be counseled regarding the possible need for a cesarean delivery depending on the extent of myometrial disruption and uterine reconstruction during surgery. Most estimates of uterine rupture rates following LM are substantially low at approximately 1% or less [21–24]. Though studies have noted that multiple/extensive uterine incisions, inadequate closure of myometrial defects, large transmural fibroids, and extensive use of electrosurgery may increase the risk of uterine rupture, its overall rarity makes it difficult to establish definitive risk factors [21,22,25]. Some experts recommend an elective cesarean section in future pregnancies with greater than 50% disruption of the myometrium during surgery [26]. Others note that any patients with prior classical or T-shaped uterine incisions, or extensive transfundal uterine surgery, should not be recommended for a trial of labor [17]. The timing of pregnancy following LM is also not well established. Studies have shown that wound healing is usually complete at 3 months postoperatively; most providers counsel patients to avoid pregnancy within the same 3–6 months following surgery [27]. There are no specific guidelines in place for this decision process. Due to the serious nature of uterine rupture in pregnancy/labor, a high index of suspicion must be maintained.

Preoperative Prophylaxis

Antibiotic prophylaxis, generally weight-based dosing of a first- or second-generation cephalosporin, is commonly used at the time of LM. This is mostly to prevent the sequelae of tubal adhesions associated with pelvic infection, which is especially important when the myomectomy is performed for infertility. Vaginal preparation prior to surgical draping is standard given the need for vaginal access and the placement of a uterine manipulator for the procedure.

Venous thromboembolic (VTE) prophylaxis should follow a risk-based approach depending on the risk factors of the patient and procedure. The "Antithrombotic Therapy and Prevention of Thrombosis, 9th ed: American College of Chest Physicians Evidence-Based Clinical Practice Guidelines," published in 2012, provides a reasonable approach for risk stratification and provision of VTE prophylaxis specifically in abdominal-pelvic surgical patients. Another useful risk-based tool is the Caprini score; though originally validated in general, vascular, and urologic surgery, extrapolation to the gynecologic patient population is reasonable [28]. If indicated, VTE prophylaxis is commonly given as a single dose of unfractionated heparin 5000 units prior to the start of surgery.

Instrumentation

The standard laparoscopy instrument set contains most of the instruments required for LM. Few studies have assessed various energy sources used for LM. The harmonic scalpel has been found to have a lower total operative time (mean 17 minutes) and EBL (mean 47 cc) when compared to conventional electrosurgery [29]. Also, the pulsed bipolar system has been associated with a lower EBL (mean 53 cc) compared to conventional electrosurgery [30]. Ultimately, the surgeon's preference and comfort level with the various energy sources should take precedence in choosing the instrumentation for the case. Additional instruments that should be prepared include a laparoscopic tenaculum to aid in providing tissue traction and countertraction for enucleation of the fibroids, a laparoscopic injection needle for vasopressin, and endoscopic bags or morcellators (see further discussion in next section) for tissue extraction. It is critical to have an operating room setup that includes all necessary instruments and devices and allows for efficient team movement (Figure 11.1).

Surgical Steps

The patient is positioned in low dorsal lithotomy position in booted support stirrups after adequate general anesthesia has been administered. To allow for adequate surgeon space at the bedside and to avoid hyperabduction of the arms, both patient arms are usually secured and tucked directly at the patient's sides with adequate padding to protect the fingers and pressure points at the wrist and elbow. Following a bimanual examination, the vagina and abdomen are both surgically prepared. A Foley catheter is then inserted, followed by a uterine manipulator (with the capability for chromopertubation if desired).

Traditionally, abdominal cavity access consists of a central or left upper quadrant 5–10 mm trocar along with two to three ancillary ports. A distance of at least 4 cm should be maintained between the primary port and the uterine fundus to allow a global view of the uterus (supraumbilical placement may be required), and the levels of the remaining accessory ports are then adjusted accordingly. Figure 11.2 depicts tumor size before surgery for proper trocar placement. If a single-site incision (SSI) approach is planned, a central 3 cm umbilical incision is used to accommodate the multiport access system with a

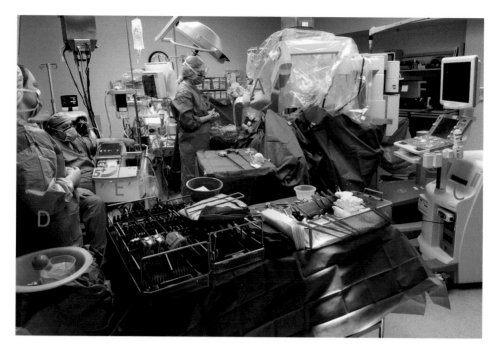

FIGURE 11.1 Operating room setup for robotic-assisted myomectomy. (A) Robot boom positioned directly over camera port trocar. (B) Bedside assistant for assistant port manipulation. (C) Bedside ultrasound if intraoperative imaging is necessary. (D) Specially trained surgical technologist. (E) Cell saver setup. (F) Capability to review relevant imaging, e.g., magnetic resonance imaging during surgery.

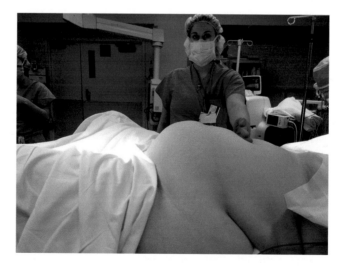

FIGURE 11.2 Clear identification of the cephalad margin of fibroid burden to guide appropriate port placement.

flexible articulating endoscope. After entry into the abdomen, a brief laparoscopic survey is performed to assess for any bowel injury at the time of entry, as well as evaluate the uterine fibroids.

A dilute vasopressin solution is usually injected at the site of planned uterine incisions (see later discussion). Uterine serosal incisions are usually placed longitudinally to facilitate LSC suturing and should avoid areas near the uterine cornua and adnexa. The total number of incisions should be minimized to preserve uterine integrity and decrease postoperative adhesion formation. Usually once the hysterotomy is made, the myometrium will retract to easily expose the fibroid capsule. The fibroid is then grasped firmly with a LSC tenaculum to create tension between the myometrium and mass. The surrounding myometrial tissue fibers are pushed away bluntly from the dissection plane to separate the fibroid capsule from the adjacent myometrium. If sharp dissection is required, care should be taken to minimize the use of electrosurgery and favor the fibroid capsule at the time of dissection to avoid extensive myometrial injury. Approximately two to four main arteries usually feed each fibroid, entering at unpredictable sites; the surgeon should be vigilant to coagulate these prior to transection whenever possible.

Once the tumors are fully enucleated, the uterine serosa is assessed to determine whether redundant tissue needs to be excised. The general principles for closure of the myometrium during an open approach apply to LM. Any endometrial defects or small deeper myometrial defects should be identified and closed first in a continuous running fashion. Of note, instillation of methylene blue (usually during chromopertubation) can be helpful to define the endometrial cavity and easily identify when the cavity has been breached. The primary incision is then closed in multiple layers (including the serosa) to improve hemostasis, prevent hematoma formation, and ensure maximum integrity of the myometrial wall. Usually, a 0-gauge delayed-absorbable suture is used; extracorporeal and intracorporeal knot tying and barbed suture are all viable options depending on surgeon skill and preference. There have been several studies that have noted reduced technical difficulty, suturing time, total operative time, and EBL with the use of barbed suture [31–33]. Video 11.1 shows some of the steps of robotic-assisted myomectomy.

VIDEO 11.1 A simple robotic-assisted myomectomy: Vasopressin injection.

URL: https://youtu.be/wOD1LpiBFwU

Tissue extraction after LM may be performed in a number of ways and has traditionally been via LSC power morcellation. However, recent concerns have emerged regarding the inadvertent dissemination of occult malignancies (such as uterine sarcomas) during power morcellation. In 2014, the U.S. Food and Drug Administration issued a report discouraging the use of LSC power morcellation for this reason [34]. Notably, the true prevalence of uterine sarcoma after myomectomies is variable, ranging from 0.1% to 0.6% [35–37]. Due to a lack of large population-based studies and to avoid denying minimally invasive surgical options for eligible patients, AAGL, the American College of Obstetricians and Gynecologists, and the Society of Gynecologic Oncology have all issued similar position statements emphasizing informed consent in lieu of complete eradication of morcellation [38–40].

Contained morcellation techniques have become more commonplace. Examples of commercially available contained extraction systems include the Alexis system from Applied Medical and the PneumoLiner system from Olympus. One method consists of manual morcellation of the fibroid inside a laparoscopic bag through an extended port incision (usually at the umbilicus). The fibroids are placed inside a large endoscopic bag. The umbilical incision is then extended to approximately 3 cm, and the opening of the bag is elevated through this incision. A self-retaining retractor is placed within the bag at the incision for ease of exposure. The fibroids are then brought up to the incision and extracted in pieces by repeated coring or wedge resections. Video 11.2 shows one of the techniques of manual morcellation using successive C-shaped incisions. Another technique involves removing the fibroids through a 3 cm posterior colpotomy. The incision may be made either LSC in the posterior cul-de-sac between the uterosacral ligaments with care to retract the nearby rectosigmoid colon, or vaginally in a fashion similar to the initial steps of a vaginal hysterectomy. The laparoscopic bag is then exteriorized against the vaginal introitus for manual morcellation. In addition to possibly lowering the risk of dissemination of occult malignancy, additional advantages of contained tissue extraction over power morcellation include anticipated lower risk of bowel injury and dissemination and development of multiple peritoneal leiomyomas as reported. The main disadvantage of contained manual morcellation is long operative time. Last, some surgeons have described the off-label use of large laparoscopic bags to create a false pneumoperitoneum in order to perform contained power morcellation. Care should be taken with the previously mentioned techniques to avoid inadvertent damage to the bag, which could lead to unintended dispersion of tissue. It should be noted that there are currently few studies regarding patient outcomes with the use of contained morcellation techniques during myomectomies.

> **VIDEO 11.2**   A simple robotic-assisted myomectomy: Uterine incision.
>
> **URL:** https://youtu.be/-vr9e1yJjFE

Additional Intraoperative Considerations

Multiple medications and methods have been assessed for decreasing EBL at the time of LM. The most robust evidence has been noted for vasopressin and misoprostol, with mean reductions in blood loss of 246 cc and 91 cc, respectively [41]. Misoprostol is usually placed rectally (400 mcg) at the time of patient positioning in the operating room, so as to not interfere with vaginal preparation for surgery. Vasopressin is standardized at 20 pressor units/mL per vial and is usually diluted at 20 units per 30–100 cc of injectable saline. Its half-life is 10–20 minutes. Vasopressin is injected at the site(s) of planned serosal incisions between the myometrium and fibroid capsule, often causing blanching at the injection sites. Needle aspiration and notifying the anesthesiologist prior to injection are vital, as a sudden increase in the patient's blood pressure may occur as a result of the medication's potent vasoconstrictor effect.

De novo adhesion formation after LM can occur in as high as 41% of cases and can adversely impact future fertility [42]. Optimal surgical technique and maintaining good hemostasis are critical for adhesion prevention. Furthermore, several barriers have been found to reduce *de novo* adhesion formation, including Interceed (oxidized regenerated cellulose) and Sepraspray/Seprafilm (chemically modified hyaluronic acid and carboxymethylcellulose) available in the United States [43–45]. These agents are applied generously at the myomectomy incision sites after they have been closed with adequate hemostasis.

Postoperative Care

Postoperative care following LM is similar to that of any major LSC surgery. The procedure is usually performed on an outpatient basis, though overnight observation in the hospital is also reasonable depending on patient comorbidities and the complexity of the case. In particular, febrile morbidity (greater than 38°C) following myomectomy is not uncommon, often attributed to myometrial incisional hematomas and inflammatory cytokines released from the myometrium. Nevertheless, the surgeon should still be vigilant regarding other more serious causes of fevers, including but not limited to pelvic infections. Return to normal activity also mirrors that of other LSC surgery; vigorous activity (heavy weight lifting, strenuous exercise) is generally delayed for 4–6 weeks following the procedure to avoid unintended complications such as incisional hernias.

Laparoscopically Assisted Myomectomy

Laparoscopically assisted myomectomy (LAM) offers a hybrid approach between LM and open abdominal myomectomy. After laparoscopic entry into the abdomen and inspection of the abdominal-pelvic cavity, a suprapubic mini-laparotomy incision (typically at the level of a standard Pfannenstiel incision) is made. A self-retaining Alexus or Mobius retractor is placed for adequate exposure through the mini-laparotomy site. The fibroid uterus can then be brought up to the level of the anterior abdominal wall or through the abdominal incision, allowing for myomectomy via a more traditional open technique. This combined approach should be considered if the fibroids are large, and extensive defects requiring significant uterine reconstruction or multilayer closure are anticipated, especially when the surgeon prefers conventional over LSC suturing. LAM can be particularly useful in cases with deep intramural fibroids where the surgeon can use direct palpation for further intraoperative surgical planning. Last, LAM provides improved visualization and exposure in cases with difficult hemostasis. In general, postoperative care and considerations for LAM procedures mirror that of LM cases.

Robotically Assisted Myomectomy

Robotically assisted LSC myomectomy (RALM) is a relatively newer minimally invasive approach that has become more commonplace in the surgical management of fibroids. Abdominal access usually consists of a central 8 or 12 mm camera port (usually 8–10 cm above the target anatomy) along with two to three ancillary 8 mm ports for the assistant robotic arms; an optional assistant side port may also be placed for additional LSC assistance at the bedside. The steps and technical considerations for myomectomy and specimen extraction are otherwise the same as those for the conventional LSC approach (Videos 11.3 through 11.8).

VIDEO 11.3   A simple robotic-assisted myomectomy: Myoma dissection (part 1).

URL: https://youtu.be/CaWyzJVwn54

VIDEO 11.4   A simple robotic-assisted myomectomy: Myoma dissection (part 2).

URL: https://youtu.be/7qznok3T3oQ

VIDEO 11.5   A simple robotic-assisted myomectomy: Myoma bed closure (part 1).

URL: https://youtu.be/L7ciy-VhZbI

VIDEO 11.6   A simple robotic-assisted myomectomy: Myoma bed closure (part 2).

URL: https://youtu.be/1k2zl7Ncxsg

VIDEO 11.7   A simple robotic-assisted myomectomy: Myoma bed closure (part 3).

URL: https://youtu.be/l7WfLeGzK-U

VIDEO 11.8   Manual morcellation of tissue in the Alexis contained-tissue extraction system.

URL: https://youtu.be/Qu0iCaOodSY

Though LSC tactile feedback is lost, robotically assisted surgery has several advantages over that of conventional LSC. It allows for three-dimensional stereoscopic view, greater dexterity with seven degrees of freedom in each of the jointed instruments, and mitigation of hand tremor, which can facilitate fibroid dissection and multilayer suturing. As such, the robotically assisted approach should be considered in more technically challenging cases, such as those with particularly large bulky fibroids, tumors involving the cervix and lower uterine segment or extending into the pelvic sidewall, or extensive pelvic adhesive disease. Overall, RALM confers similar patient care benefits as those of LM when compared to traditional open myomectomy, including lower blood loss and less need for blood transfusions, shorter hospital stays, and lower perioperative complication rates [46]. Figure 11.3 shows the sequential steps of robotic-assisted myomectomy. The common disadvantage for robotic surgery is the financial cost, including higher hospital/professional charges, and hospital reimbursement rates.

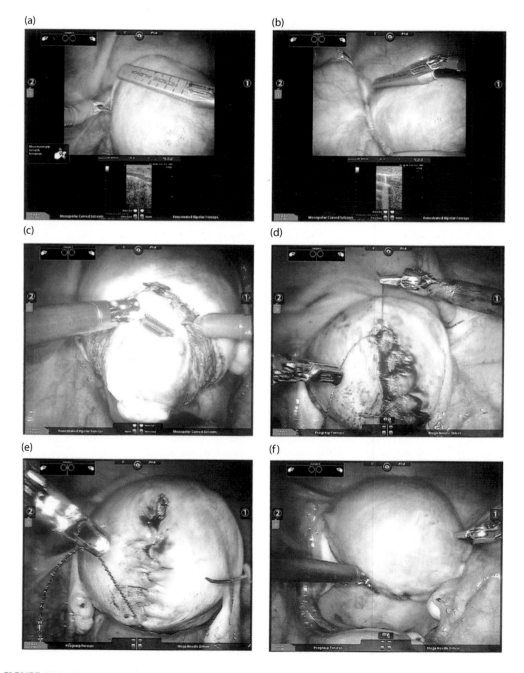

FIGURE 11.3 Sequential steps of robotic-assisted myomectomy. (a,b) Intraoperative ultrasound guidance (note live ultrasound images on lower part of panel). (c) Initial incision and dissection of fibroid. (d) Myometrial suturing to close fibroid bed. (e) Baseball suture incorporating serosa. (f) Completed closure of incision.

Intraoperative Ultrasound Guidance

A useful adjunct to LM is the intraoperative use of ultrasound guidance to locate intramural/submucosal fibroids for more complete resection and accurate delineation of endometrial cavity. One of the disadvantages of LM, compared to the conventional open approach, is the inability to directly palpate the uterus to locate various fibroids for resection. Even with adequate preoperative evaluation, it can sometimes be difficult to accurately locate deeper and smaller fibroids, which can lead to misplaced uterine incisions, in turn causing increased blood loss, operating time, and reduced myometrial integrity. Furthermore, residual myomas may lead to increased rates of symptomatic recurrence, reoperation, and infertility.

Several case reports and studies have commented on the feasibility and effectiveness of LSC, robotic-assisted, and traditional transvaginal intraoperative ultrasound guidance at the time of LM [47–49]. For LSC ultrasound guidance, the ultrasound probe is inserted through a LSC port and positioned intra-abdominally through LSC manipulation. The probe is brought in contact with the uterus to scan for fibroids that would otherwise not be easily localized. At our institution, we use the ProSound Alpha 7 system (Hitachi Healthcare) and the corresponding linear probes available for both robotic (UST-5550-R) and traditional LSC (UST-5550) configurations. The TilePro multi-input display allows combined real-time views of both operative and ultrasound images for both the surgeon and the operating room team. Transvaginal ultrasonography is widely available with lower cost and can be used alone or in conjunction with LSC ultrasound guidance for precise localization of fibroids [47,48]. Notably, it has been shown that LSC and transvaginal ultrasound guidance during LM can aid in the resection of significantly smaller residual fibroids with a trend toward decreased fibroid recurrence rates [48]. Figures 11.1, 11.3, and 11.4 demonstrate the integration of intraoperative ultrasound into robotic-assisted myomectomy.

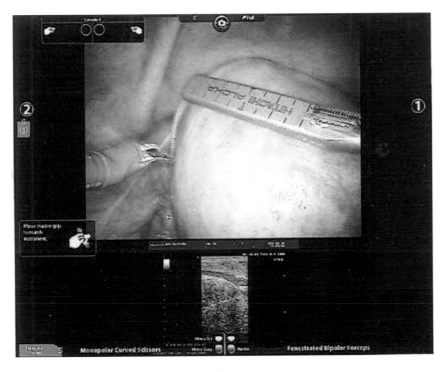

FIGURE 11.4 Intraoperative ultrasound use during robotic-assisted myomectomy. Please note the the TilePro function of the da Vinci Surgical System that allows the multi-input simultaneous display of the robotic camera (top panel) and the ultrasound image (lower panel) at the surgeon console view.

REFERENCES

1. Sizzi O, Rossetti A, Malzoni M et al. Italian multicenter study on complications of laparoscopic myomectomy. *J Minim Invasive Gynecol.* 2007;14(4):453–62.
2. Donnez J and Dolmans MM. Uterine fibroid management: From the present to the future. *Hum Reprod Update.* 2016;22(6):665–86.
3. Chen CC and Falcone T. Robotic gynecologic surgery: Past, present, and future. *Clin Obstet Gynecol.* 2009;52(3):335–43.
4. Lee J and Spies J. Management options for uterine fibroids. In: Geschwind J and Dake M (eds) *Abrams' Angiography: Interventional Radiology.* 3rd ed. Philadelphia, PA: Lippincott Williams & Wilkins; 2014, pp. 239–45.
5. Rutgers JL, Spong CY, Sinow R, and Heiner J. Leuprolide acetate treatment and myoma arterial size. *Obstet Gynecol.* 1995;86(3):386–8.
6. Chen I, Motan T, and Kiddoo D. Gonadotropin-releasing hormone agonist in laparoscopic myomectomy: Systematic review and meta-analysis of randomized controlled trials. *J Minim Invasive Gynecol.* 2011;18(3):303–9.
7. Palomba S, Pellicano M, Affinito P, Di Carlo C, Zullo F, and Nappi C. Effectiveness of short-term administration of tibolone plus gonadotropin-releasing hormone analogue on the surgical outcome of laparoscopic myomectomy. *Fertil Steril.* 2001;75(2):429–33.
8. Donnez J, Tomaszewski J, Vazquez F et al. Ulipristal acetate versus leuprolide acetate for uterine fibroids. *N Engl J Med.* 2012;366(5):421–32.
9. Leone Roberti Maggiore U, Scala C, Venturini PL, and Ferrero S. Preoperative treatment with letrozole in patients undergoing laparoscopic myomectomy of large uterine myomas: A prospective non-randomized study. *Eur J Obstet Gynecol Reprod Biol.* 2014;181:157–62.
10. Holub Z, Mara M, Kuzel D, Jabor A, Maskova J, and Eim J. Pregnancy outcomes after uterine artery occlusion: Prospective multicentric study. *Fertil Steril.* 2008;90(5):1886–91.
11. Goldman KN, Hirshfeld-Cytron JE, Pavone ME, Thomas AP, Vogelzang RL, and Milad MP. Uterine artery embolization immediately preceding laparoscopic myomectomy. *Int J Gynaecol Obstet.* 2012;116(2):105–8.
12. Mara M, Maskova J, Fucikova Z, Kuzel D, Belsan T, and Sosna O. Midterm clinical and first reproductive results of a randomized controlled trial comparing uterine fibroid embolization and myomectomy. *Cardiovasc Intervent Radiol.* 2008;31(1):73–85.
13. Hovsepian DM, Siskin GP, Bonn J et al. Quality improvement guidelines for uterine artery embolization for symptomatic leiomyomata. *J Vasc Interv Radiol.* 2009;20(7 suppl):S193–9.
14. Worthington-Kirsch RL. Uterine artery embolization: State of the art. *Semin Intervent Radiol.* 2004;21(1): 37–42.
15. Pron G, Mocarski E, Bennett J et al. Pregnancy after uterine artery embolization for leiomyomata: The Ontario multicenter trial. *Obstet Gynecol.* 2005;105(1):67–76.
16. Dutton S, Hirst A, McPherson K, Nicholson T, and Maresh M. A UK multicentre retrospective cohort study comparing hysterectomy and uterine artery embolisation for the treatment of symptomatic uterine fibroids (HOPEFUL study): Main results on medium-term safety and efficacy. *BJOG.* 2007;114(11):1340–51.
17. American College of Obstetricians and Gynecologists. ACOG practice bulletin. alternatives to hysterectomy in the management of leiomyomas. *Obstet Gynecol.* 2008, Reaffirmed 2016;112(2 Pt 1):387–400.
18. Radosa MP, Owsianowski Z, Mothes A et al. Long-term risk of fibroid recurrence after laparoscopic myomectomy. *Eur J Obstet Gynecol Reprod Biol.* 2014;180:35–9.
19. Doridot V, Dubuisson JB, Chapron C, Fauconnier A, and Babaki-Fard K. Recurrence of leiomyomata after laparoscopic myomectomy. *J Am Assoc Gynecol Laparosc.* 2001;8(4):495–500.
20. Nezhat FR, Roemisch M, Nezhat CH, Seidman DS, and Nezhat CR. Recurrence rate after laparoscopic myomectomy. *J Am Assoc Gynecol Laparosc.* 1998;5(3):237–40.
21. Koo YJ, Lee JK, Lee YK et al. Pregnancy outcomes and risk factors for uterine rupture after laparoscopic myomectomy: A single-center experience and literature review. *J Minim Invasive Gynecol.* 2015;22(6):1022–8.
22. Parker WH, Einarsson J, Istre O, and Dubuisson JB. Risk factors for uterine rupture after laparoscopic myomectomy. *J Minim Invasive Gynecol.* 2010;17(5):551–4.

23. Gambacorti-Passerini Z, Gimovsky AC, Locatelli A, and Berghella V. Trial of labor after myomectomy and uterine rupture: A systematic review. *Acta Obstet Gynecol Scand.* 2016;95(7):724–34.

24. Claeys J, Hellendoom I, Hamerlynch T, Bosteels J, and Weters S. The risk of uterine rupture after myomectomy: A systematic review of the literature and meta-analysis. *Gynecol Surg.* 2014;1(197):197–206.

25. Bernardi TS, Radosa MP, Weisheit A et al. Laparoscopic myomectomy: A 6-year follow-up single-center cohort analysis of fertility and obstetric outcome measures. *Arch Gynecol Obstet.* 2014;290(1):87–91.

26. Alessandri F, Lijoi D, Mistrangelo E, Ferrero S, and Ragni N. Randomized study of laparoscopic versus mini-laparotomic myomectomy for uterine myomas. *J Minim Invasive Gynecol.* 2006;13(2):92–7.

27. Darwish AM, Nasr AM, and El-Nashar DA. Evaluation of postmyomectomy uterine scar. *J Clin Ultrasound.* 2005;33(4):181–6.

28. Gould MK, Garcia DA, Wren SM et al. Prevention of VTE in nonorthopedic surgical patients: Antithrombotic therapy and prevention of thrombosis, 9th ed: American College of Chest Physicians evidence-based clinical practice guidelines. *Chest.* 2012;141(2 suppl):e227S–77S.

29. Litta P, Fantinato S, Calonaci F et al. A randomized controlled study comparing harmonic versus electrosurgery in laparoscopic myomectomy. *Fertil Steril.* 2010;94(5):1882–6.

30. Su H, Han CM, Wang CJ, Lee CL, and Soong YK. Comparison of the efficacy of the pulsed bipolar system and conventional electrosurgery in laparoscopic myomectomy—A retrospective matched control study. *Taiwan J Obstet Gynecol.* 2011;50(1):25–8.

31. Song T, Kim TJ, Kim WY, and Lee SH. Comparison of barbed suture versus traditional suture in laparoendoscopic single-site myomectomy. *Eur J Obstet Gynecol Reprod Biol.* 2015;185:99–102.

32. Tulandi T and Einarsson JI. The use of barbed suture for laparoscopic hysterectomy and myomectomy: A systematic review and meta-analysis. *J Minim Invasive Gynecol.* 2014;21(2):210–6.

33. Alessandri F, Remorgida V, Venturini PL, and Ferrero S. Unidirectional barbed suture versus continuous suture with intracorporeal knots in laparoscopic myomectomy: A randomized study. *J Minim Invasive Gynecol.* 2010;17(6):725–9.

34. U.S. Food and Drug Administration. *Laparoscopic Power Morcellators.* U.S. Food and Drug Administration website. Accessed June 2020. https://www.fda.gov/medical-devices/surgery-devices/laparoscopic-power-morcellators#:~:text=The%20FDA%20recommends%20health%20care,or%20hysterectomy%20for%20uterine%20fibroids. Updated Feb 2020.

35. Lieng M, Berner E, and Busund B. Risk of morcellation of uterine leiomyosarcomas in laparoscopic supracervical hysterectomy and laparoscopic myomectomy, a retrospective trial including 4791 women. *J Minim Invasive Gynecol.* 2015;22(3):410–4.

36. Wright JD, Tergas AI, Burke WM et al. Uterine pathology in women undergoing minimally invasive hysterectomy using morcellation. *JAMA.* 2014;312(12):1253–5.

37. Tan-Kim J, Hartzell KA, Reinsch CS et al. Uterine sarcomas and parasitic myomas after laparoscopic hysterectomy with power morcellation. *Am J Obstet Gynecol.* 2015;212(5):594.e1–10.

38. Goff BA. SGO not soft on morcellation: Risks and benefits must be weighed. *Lancet Oncol.* 2014;15(4):e148.

39. AAGL Advancing Minimally Invasive Gynecology Worldwide. AAGL practice report: Morcellation during uterine tissue extraction. *J Minim Invasive Gynecol.* 2014;21(4):517–30.

40. American College of Obstetricians and Gynecologists. *Power morcellation and occult malignancy in gynecologic surgery.* American College of Obstetricians and Gynecologists Special Report. 2014.

41. Kongnyuy EJ, van den Broek N, and Wiysonge CS. A systematic review of randomized controlled trials to reduce hemorrhage during myomectomy for uterine fibroids. *Int J Gynaecol Obstet.* 2008;100(1):4–9.

42. Dubuisson JB, Fauconnier A, Chapron C, Kreiker G, and Norgaard C. Second look after laparoscopic myomectomy. *Hum Reprod.* 1998;13(8):2102–6.

43. Tinelli A, Malvasi A, Guido M et al. Adhesion formation after intracapsular myomectomy with or without adhesion barrier. *Fertil Steril.* 2011;95(5):1780–5.

44. Fossum GT, Silverberg KM, Miller CE, Diamond MP, and Holmdahl L. Gynecologic use of Sepraspray adhesion barrier for reduction of adhesion development after laparoscopic myomectomy: A pilot study. *Fertil Steril.* 2011;96(2):487–91.

45. Ahmad G, O'Flynn H, Hindocha A, and Watson A. Barrier agents for adhesion prevention after gynaecological surgery. *Cochrane Database Syst Rev.* 2015;(4):CD000475.

46. Iavazzo C, Mamais I, and Gkegkes ID. Robotic assisted vs laparoscopic and/or open myomectomy: Systematic review and meta-analysis of the clinical evidence. *Arch Gynecol Obstet.* 2016;294(1):5–17.

47. Lin PC, Thyer A, and Soules MR. Intraoperative ultrasound during a laparoscopic myomectomy. *Fertil Steril.* 2004;81(6):1671–4.
48. Shimanuki H, Takeuchi H, Kikuchi I, Kumakiri J, and Kinoshita K. Effectiveness of intraoperative ultrasound in reducing recurrent fibroids during laparoscopic myomectomy. *J Reprod Med.* 2006;51(9):683–8.
49. Paul P, Ahluvalia D, Narasimhan D et al. Intraoperative transvaginal sonography: A novel approach for localization of deeper myomas during laparoscopic myomectomy. *Gynecol Surg.* 2015;12(4):303–8.

Index